Combat-Ready Kitchen

CURRENT

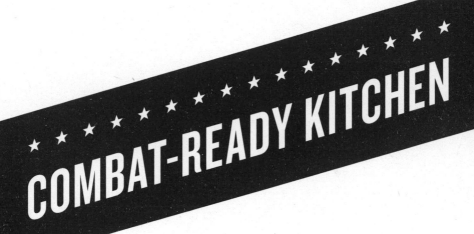

★ ★ ★ ★ ★ ★ ★ ★ ★ ★
COMBAT-READY KITCHEN

How the U.S. Military Shapes
the Way You Eat

Anastacia Marx de Salcedo

CURRENT

CURRENT
An imprint of Penguin Random House LLC
375 Hudson Street
New York, New York 10014
penguin.com

ISBN 978-1-59184-597-3

Printed in the United States of America
10   9   8   7   6   5   4   3   2   1

Set in Warnock Pro with Knockout and Helvetica Neue
Designed by Daniel Lagin

For My Girls

———————

Se hace camino al andar

—Antonio Machado

Contents

Combat-Ready Kitchen

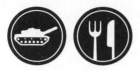

For about three days when we were in Kuwait in 2003 and U.S. forces were advancing into Iraq, the sirens would go off, and we'd have to put on our gas masks and our MOPP* gear and get into our bunker. Saddam was sending what we thought were Scuds with chemical weapons at us, but actually turned out to be smaller missiles. We'd have to wait for the all clear, which would sometimes take a long time.

We really shouldn't have been eating in the bunker, but sometimes we'd get hungry, so we'd eat an MRE.† Usually only one person had one, so we were sharing between everyone. There were probably ten of us in there. It's a concrete bunker where you can't stand up, you can't really sit down, you're sitting on a sandbag, and you're leaning forward because your head's hitting the ceiling. Everyone's wearing flak jackets, environmental suits, and a gas mask and helmet. So we'd pass around an MRE, take off the gas mask for ten seconds, and grab a bite of, like, Salisbury steak. And then we'd put our gas masks back on and pass it over to the next guy.

I remember when the guy pulled out the MRE. Everyone sitting in there is so hungry, we haven't eaten in hours, and so when he offered to share,

---

* Mission Oriented Protective Posture.
† Meal, Ready-to-Eat.

we were all really happy. It was kind of like a bonding moment. We knew that we didn't have any control over what was going to happen, and we were all breaking the rules by taking our gas masks off and eating when we shouldn't be. It brought us all to the same place. We were all stuck there. It didn't matter whether you were a private or a master sergeant, you were stuck there in that bunker.

—DJ, Corporal, United States Marine Corps, Al Jabar, Kuwait, and Al Asad, Iraq, 2003–6

Chapter 1

UNPACKING YOUR CHILD'S LUNCH BOX

Dirty, hungry, uncomfortable, and scared. Most of us can't imagine what it's like to eat under the circumstances that DJ and his squad did. The experiences of war, if an American constant during the twentieth and twenty-first centuries, seem remote to the average person. And we certainly don't imagine that the entrée the soldiers shared—a several-years-old beef patty with brown sauce in a laminated plastic-and-foil pouch—has anything to do with the food that fills our refrigerators, cupboards, and shelves. But it does.

★ ★ ★

I'VE ALWAYS BEEN A PASSIONATE HOME COOK, one who read recipe books in bed like novels, preferred browsing at an ethnic grocer's or a farmers' market to shoe shopping, and reliably created magical dinners where people lingered long into the night, talking, drinking, and nibbling until there were no leftovers. Although my own mother was indifferent to the matter, as a child I silently apprenticed myself to the three best cooks I knew—my Yankee grandmother, my Sephardic New Yorker grandfather, and my Mexican friend's mother—sidling into their kitchens and absorbing by osmosis their doings. At the age of seven, I proudly presented my parents with my first creation: "spiced eggs" scrambled with every single flavoring from the rack. By the time I was in my midtwenties, I had read everything in M. F. K. Fisher's oeuvre, and, inspired by—but not following—the thousands of recipes I'd mentally collected, cosseted my college boyfriend nightly with delectable little suppers prepared just for him.

When the new millennium rolled around, I'd acquired a husband—from Cuba, in Ecuador—and become a mother, which only strengthened my resolve to concoct everything from scratch, even pancakes, whipped cream, and mac 'n' cheese. I spent an inordinate amount of time provisioning, trucking out to farms weekly for two separate community-supported agriculture locations, one for meat and the other for vegetables; ladling bulk items into flimsy plastic bags at my local co-op; and scouring Asian, Latin, and Middle Eastern groceries for exotic produce, spices, specialty meats, and condiments. Regardless of how much my children pleaded, I refused to stop at McDonald's on car trips. I even became a leader of Boston's Slow Food convivium, finding time to organize a cocktail party featuring local Brazilian culture, teach Boston schoolkids how to make their own vegetable burritos, and celebrate the humble bean with a hundred-plus-person potluck and a reading by a renowned food historian. It was exhausting. It was fun. And it made me feel good—proudly conscientious. As many do, I fervently believed that it was important to cook, that it brought together my family in a vital ritual, that the dishes I produced were healthier and more satisfying, and that it was part of a human heritage that embedded us in the world, both past and present.

Which is why, when it came to school, I made the extra effort to pack my daughters a nutritious, homemade meal. I could have signed them up for the school meals program, where blue-capped cafeteria ladies grimly plop onto trays a hot entrée, such as the dreaded sloppy joe, insipid pizza, or turkey with gravy; a vegetable (canned peas/green beans/corn); a slightly rancid carton of milk; and Jell-O, fruit cocktail, or a mealy apple. (The menu has improved slightly in recent years—wheat instead of white buns, no dessert, and some scraggly schoolyard-grown broccoli.) But an involved parent, a mother who cares about what her children eat, makes their lunches herself. To do so, I relaxed my stance against processed foods, which, I have to confess, had long ago snuck into my home, first with my husband and eventually, under the duress of relentless lobbying, with me. Armed with child-pleasing supplies culled from the shelves of the supermarket, I set about my task. Into the nylon carrier with its cunningly zipped insulated vinyl compartments and controlled-atmosphere Tupperware, I put Goldfish, an energy bar, a juice pouch, and a sandwich. This last I'd assembled with my own two hands: soft twelve-grain bread, turkey ham, and a slice of American cheese swathed in Saran wrap. A couple of baby carrots and some grapes to round things out. I put the two lunch boxes in the refrigerator, poured myself a fishbowl of Shiraz, and went to bed, confident that I'd done my best by them.

Or had I?

As my children had gotten older, I'd started a side career as a food writer. After a few pieces about Latin American cooking—*fiestas de Pascua* (Easter), Ecuadorian soups, street food—I found myself increasingly drawn to writing not about home cooking, my own or that of others, but about the industrial foodstuffs that I, with annoyance, accepted as staples in my pantry. First off the block was that insidious impostor Annie's mac 'n' cheese, pretending to be more wholesome than it was: I read the label very carefully, and it turned out to have practically the same components as the neon-orange standby, Kraft's. The Internet exploded, mostly with vitriolic responses by parents defending their reliance on "the Bunny" and his wares as a decision that was somehow healthier than buying an almost identical nutrition-free product from a major conglomerate.

I had found my topic.

My next piece, on breakfast cereal, led me deeper into the real world of food processing. I dug into the history of our archetypical carbohydrate and read up on its modern-day production, schooling myself in the functioning of that mainstay of manufacturing, the extruder, which uses a screw or a ram to push metal, plastic, ceramics, and food through a long chamber, where it is heated by friction and pressure (and, in some cases, electrical heat) and then forced through a die. In addition to cereal, extruders are used to create many other starchy foods, including pastas, pet foods, and snack foods. The latter can be hollow and then filled, or puffed by exposing them to reduced pressure on exiting. (Cheetos, one of the first extruder-produced junk foods, are fabricated this way.) Extrusion cooking requires little moisture, so the resulting foods are dry and last a long time without refrigeration. As I delved further into the ideas, ingredients, and technology, I began to see that to understand how industrial food was made, I'd need to have a good grasp of physics, chemistry, and biology. Little did I know where that would lead me.

I took my newfound food-science research skills and applied them to children's lunch boxes. I was in for an unpleasant surprise: by no measure—environmental, nutritional, or freshness—did the meal I'd diligently "prepared" for my children surpass that of the much-maligned school lunch. I compared the Goldfish, energy bar, sandwich, carrots, and grapes with a typical cafeteria meal—chicken tenderloins with sauce, brown rice, cooked frozen carrots, canned peaches in syrup, and milk. The school lunch blew the brown bag out of the water. Many of the ingredients in the cafeteria food come in enormous sacks and cans, minimizing packaging waste, and were prepared in large quantities, cutting the fuel used per serving to almost zero. The refuse from your child's lunch box, on the other hand, would have sent your grandparents or great-grandparents into cardiac arrest: a laminated pouch from the juice, packaging from the Goldfish and energy bar, plastic wrap in which you put the sandwich, and a paper napkin, not to mention the wrappers from the sandwich ingredients. While the school meal wasn't exactly a paragon of nutrition—it clocked in at 600 calories, 17.5 grams of fat (3.5 grams saturated), 57 milligrams of cholesterol, and 1,131 milligrams of sodium—it beat out my repast, which had a total of 643 calories, 20.1 grams of fat (8.5 grams saturated), 50 milligrams of cholesterol, 994 milligrams of sodium, and 38 grams of sugar (the school lunch didn't report sugar). Even more devastating, the cafeteria meal, which is largely concocted of frozen raw or partially cooked ingredients, was much closer to food in its natural state. Sure, the strips of chicken coated with bread crumbs are Tyson's; the cryonic carrot coins have traveled three thousand miles from California's Central Valley; and the rice was par-boiled and plumped up in an industrial steamer. But overall, this meal had fewer ingredients and the animal and plant tissues of its components were still recognizable.

How did that compare with my offering, put together with the best intentions in the intimacy of my own kitchen? I already knew that the Goldfish, energy bar, and juice pouch had long shelf lives. It's one of the reasons we parents buy them. The facts that such foods can be stored at room temperature for an extended duration, are easy to carry and hard to destroy, are wrapped in single servings, and are eagerly scarfed up by children make them the leitmotif of the weekday lunch. I let my guilt at including these admittedly overprocessed items be assuaged by the fact that they were just the backdrop to the main act, made the night before from ingredients I myself had excavated from the refrigerator and bread box. Except that the turkey ham, formed from poultry protein that's been mechanically separated from the bone, tumbled with salt, sugar, preservatives, and plenty of water, then cooked, is also strangely long-lived, lasting for up to two weeks. Ditto the slice of white or orange (a touch of annatto gives it its cheery hue) American cheese, which can be kept for a month. Even the bread, the daily freshness of which was so important that for thousands of years chronically sleep-deprived men spent their nights shoveling dough into and hot loaves out of village ovens, is now long in the tooth—treated with high-fructose corn syrup and starch-snacking enzymes, it goes weeks without changing taste. Together the items in my "homemade" lunch were probably older than my kids.

In early 2011, I wrote a piece saying as much for a PBS blog where I was a contributor. My point: the components of the brown bag's center-piece foodstuff, far from being fresh and healthy, were positively geriatric, tricked up to appear youthful and brimming with artificial and possibly harmful ingredients. (I may have made an unfortunate comparison to Donatella Versace.) But I'd learned something else in my research, something that I didn't put in the piece, a puzzling nugget of information that I hoarded for later. As I untangled the thread of extended shelf life for both the turkey ham and the soft "whole grain" bread in my sandwich, at their origins I found attributions to work done by an obscure U.S. Army base, the Natick Soldier Systems Center. What was it, and what was its relation to the processed foods we Americans eat every day?

Those questions became a book proposal. Soon after we sent it out, my agent called with a deal from a Penguin imprint, which I promptly Googled for its specialty. Science? A science publisher wanted my book? But then I realized, yes, of course, the topic, how the military constructs the underpinnings of industrial food, was all about science and technology. The last science course I'd taken was rocks for jocks at Columbia, but I gamely rolled up my sleeves and waded in. Over the next two and a half years, I talked to soldiers, scientists, and historians; I poked around in the Natick Center's equipment-jammed laboratories; I combed over old meeting notes and reports; I spelunked declassified Department of Defense documents and the U.S. Patent and Trademark database. And I probably became the only regular nonprofessional reader of publications such as *Cereal Chemistry, Comprehensive Reviews in Food Science and Food Safety, Journal of Dairy Science, Nebraska Swine Report, Applied and Environmental Microbiology, Journal of Polymer Science,* and *Toxicological Sciences,* including, at times, their back issues to the early 1930s.

The answers to my questions about the Natick Center, contained in these pages, floored me. The reason we send our children to school with heavily processed, hermetically sealed convenience foods isn't (only) that big corporations, preying on our hectic lifestyle and relief that there's *something* the little dears will eat, have created these items, most of them manufactured from the cheapest calories around, to maximize profits— your kid's health and the planet's be damned. No, it's far worse than that. Your child's lunch isn't healthful, fresh, or environmentally sound because it wasn't designed for children. It was designed for soldiers. Almost all of the foodstuffs, or the key technologies used in producing them, originated with the U.S. military in the creation of combat rations. In developing them, the army was seeking some of the very same qualities we do in putting together our children's out-of-home midday meal:

portability, ease of preparation, extended shelf life at room temperature, affordability, and appeal to even the least adventurous eaters. In other words, we've got our children chowing down like special ops.

It's time to unpack your child's lunch box and unravel the secret military past of just about everything in it.

Chapter 2

AMERICAN FOOD SYSTEM, CENTRAL COMMAND, PART ONE

I'm not at liberty to divulge the top secret way I got my embarrassingly old and dented Camry to the Natick Soldier Center gatehouse, but suffice it to say there are various uniformed men and a lot of concrete barriers involved. Once inside, my car is checked for improvised explosive devices and I'm met by Lieutenant Colonel David Accetta, a creased-pants, crushing-handshake kind of guy who signs his e-mails "All the Way! David." He opens the passenger-side door and slides in.

"Buckle up," he commands, swiveling so I can see the two scars crisscrossing his face as if he'd been run over by an M1 Abrams tank. "This is a federal facility, and we're strict." I'm barely going five miles per hour and it's a parking lot, but I do what he says.

The U.S. Army Natick Soldier Research, Development and Engineering Center, a handful of low buildings scattered over seventy-eight acres in a nondescript Boston suburb, could be just another second-tier office park. The Combat Feeding Directorate, one of seven research centers on the site, is toward the back, in an H-shaped, teal-and-aqua-striped building surrounded—like that drive-you-crazy neighbor's house— by slightly rusting vehicles, except in this case there's a Humvee, a camouflage-tarped assault kitchen, a shower/laundry unit, and a ten-by-twenty-foot steel box with a containerized chapel.

As Hollywood is to movies, as Nashville is to country music, and as New York City is to the publishing industry, the Natick Center is to the processed foods that form the bedrock of the American diet. It's where they invented energy bars, restructured meat, nonstaling bread, and instant coffee. And today, in a marathon eight-hour visit, I'll witness how the U.S. Army designs the rations that—reformulated and repackaged—line our pantry shelves and fill our refrigerators. I've breached the secret beating heart of the industrial food system.

The American soldier stationed abroad eats a diet almost as varied as we do here at home. Sparing no expense, the Department of Defense (DOD), via a multibillion-dollar, sole-source "prime vendor" contract (the companies are often owned, at least in part, by former military members and headquartered abroad),[1] ships in fresh meat, dairy, and produce from nearby allics. The cost of these perishables is almost double their stateside price tag due to the difficulty of transport over ambush-prone roads and to remote areas with little infrastructure. The fresh supplies are combined with stockpiled staples and preserved items purchased directly from American food conglomerates such as ConAgra, Sara Lee, and Perdue for made-from-scratch meals in the garrison mess halls. (Well, as from-scratch as a modern American meal ever is, that is to say, prepared by opening bags, boxes, bottles, and cans.) And should our warrior ever crave an Ultimate Cheese Lover's Pizza, a Triple Whopper, or the Colonel's Crispy Strips, she can visit the fast-food stands that are now a fixture on foreign military bases.

But what about on the front line, when the soldier is engaged in activities that are, of course, the real reason he's stationed thousands of miles from home, sleeping fitfully in a tent, alternately bored or adrenaline-charged and fearful? Performing a function check on his M16. Searching civilian vehicles at a checkpoint. Digging foxholes. Guiding down a "bird" to an improvised landing strip. Warriors in the field may be there for days on end, their souped-up metabolisms burning up to 4,200 calories over twenty-four hours, but the brutal business of kill or be killed hardly lends itself to sit-down meals. Enter the Natick Center. Their contribution to the army's feeding strategy is reserved for a single occasion: combat. The graze-'n'-raze product line includes the Meal, Ready-to-Eat (MRE); First Strike Ration; Unitized Group Ration (UGR); Meal, Cold Weather, and Food Packet, Long Range Patrol; and the Modular Operational Ration Enhancement (MORE). Each has been laboriously engineered and manufactured on American soil to deliver an optimal nutritional payload to soldiers half a world and several years away.

Lieutenant Colonel Accetta escorts me into the Combat Feeding Directorate building. Immediately to the left is the Warrior Café, a small meeting room stuffed with rations memorabilia—Civil War hardtack, a jaw-breaking square cracker poked full of holes to ensure even baking; World War II C-rats in gold-lacquered cans with their inevitable companion, the P-38 can opener; the similar Korean and Vietnam War–era canned Meal, Combat, Individuals; tiny vials of synthetic smells; and a wall case full of elderly bakery products. Kathy-Lynn Evangelos, second in charge at the directorate; Lauren Oleksyk, a food scientist; and two Iraq War vets, tall and lanky Corporal Evan Bick and short and broad Jeff Sisto, await us. Introductions are made all around and then eyes snap back to Evangelos, the power center. She flashes the tight smile of someone due elsewhere five minutes ago and launches into her boilerplate overview of the Combat Feeding Program.

"Our shelf life is three years at eighty degrees because combat rations are a war-stopper and protected by Congress. When you go to war, you've got to bring your beans and your bullets. And those beans have to be shelf stable, high quality, and ready to go. When you talk to food technologists in the commercial sector, they'll ask us what our shelf life is and we'll tell them and they'll be in shock," she says, rattling off a list of the typical research activities at a private company: an umpteenth flavor for a product line; a new, giant cookie sandwich; fanciful cracker shapes. But when it comes down to the nitty-gritty—getting those things to last for three, six, or nine months without spoiling or going stale: "Shelf life is the challenge—and the experts are here at Natick."

Evangelos is already eyeing her watch—her five minutes are up. But I have to ask a question, the one that, although they don't know it, is the real reason for my visit: How often do the Natick Center's inventions get adapted by the private sector? "We don't necessarily want to develop things that are militarily unique, so we're really anxious when it comes to technology transfer," she explains. "If it's something new and innovative, we're not going to develop it here, use it here, and that's the end of it. We need to have the commercial sector embrace anything new that comes out of this program." (Later I ask the eminent food scientist and former *Journal of Food Science* editor Daryl Lund the same thing. His answer is more explicit: "If an emergency arises, they need to be able to go to those companies and say, 'Hey, you have a processing line that produces these kinds of foods for the consumer, but now we need you to convert it to produce these same kinds of foods for the military.'") Spiel done, Evangelos excuses herself, bustles down the hall, and disappears through two swinging doors that lead to another wing of the building.

Immediately, the two vets, corporals Bick and Sisto, heave a cardboard box full of rations onto the table. "Ready to taste?"

The rations, tan bundles made of heavy-grade thermoplastic polyolefin, are easy to toss in a rucksack. They weigh 1⅝ pounds and are just about the size of a brick. Inside each shrink-wrapped package are close to twenty separate items: two transparent plastic bags, one for beverages and the other for the flameless heater; several three- or four-layer pouches made of foil, polyethylene, nylon, and polyester that encase an entrée, pastry items, crackers, breads, cereals, and spreads; cylindrical plastic packets of coffee and a Kool-Aid-like beverage; paper packets of salt and sugar; a plastic spoon; a packet of nondairy creamer; a matchbook; two Chiclets in white-and-red cellophane; and a tightly folded square of toilet paper. (After their meal, soldiers burn or bury all trash.)

The guys are nudging toward me what I'm guessing they think I'll like, Menu 14, Spicy Penne with Vegetarian Sausage, and Menu 23,

Chicken Pesto Pasta, but as an MRE neophyte, I'm going for the gusto. I choose an American classic: Menu 18, Beef Patty, which at 1,200 calories and chock-full of glucose is calibrated to the metabolism of an Ironman triathlete. It's also been sitting at room temperature for two years. I resolutely rip open the package and start with the most familiar item, Combos, or rather crispy tubes of dough filled with gooey processed cheese. They're very tasty, and I finish the bag. The whole wheat bread "snack," on the other hand, can't be much of an improvement on the aforementioned hardtack. And the pièce de résistance, a hamburger heated in one of the transparent bags by a magnesium, salt, iron, and water chemical reaction, veers alarmingly toward not being fit for human consumption.

"Delicious," I say.

Next on the tasting menu is the First Strike Ration, which, as Corporal Bick explains, is "designed for a grazing mentality." It was formally introduced in 2007, after it was found that soldiers were stripping MREs of their snackier elements to make them easier to carry into battle, which, unfortunately, also stripped the meals of their nutritional value. The package, which contains 3,900 calories, enough for an entire day, includes, among other things, a three-year shelf-stable sandwich; an energy bar, originally called the HooAH! bar, in honor of the army call used to affirm or motivate soldiers; and, my personal favorite, caffeinated gum. I pop two pieces into my mouth.

"Careful," says Lieutenant Colonel Accetta. "Those will give you a stomachache." Then he gives a half wave. "Excuse me. I have some work to do. I'll check in on you later." He strides off toward the back of the building and through the swinging doors.

"Would you like to see the food lab?" asks Lauren Oleksyk, the leader of the Food Processing, Engineering and Technology Team. She's your archetypical girl-nerd: slight, medium height, dressed to deflect attention. A career food scientist, she doesn't bother to provide synonyms for words like exothermic reaction or thermal stabilization.

The food lab is the size of a small airplane hangar—spotless stainless steel counters and sinks, gleaming gauges and valves—and practically lifeless, except for three women standing off to the left, talking and laughing as they flatten out rounds of dough, stuff them, and crimp the edges closed. It could be the annual empanada blowout at Tía Elena's, except instead of rolling pins, they wield steel rods encased in silicone padding. And instead of aprons, they're wearing lab coats and hairnets. They are food technologists Jacqueline LeBlanc, Danielle Anderson, and Sydney Walker. Today they're working on the shelf-stable sandwich, perfecting a new sausage-and-cheese flavor to add to the existing lineup of pepperoni and chicken barbecue.

"The secret is the marinade," says LeBlanc in that conspiratorial tone cooks get when they're about to share a treasured recipe. I lean forward, expecting some piquant cousin of a traditional barbecue sauce. "Rice syrup and glycerol to bring down the water activity of the sausage. Artificial sausage flavor because anything that's supposed to last such a long time will lose a little flavor. And we're trying two different acidulants in the meat. I'm just hoping it doesn't affect the flavor too much." Increasing its acidity helps to preserve the meat, because most pathogenic bacteria can't reproduce at a pH lower than 4.6.

Recipes published in cookbooks and magazines and on Web sites are usually developed and tested over a period of days or weeks. Formulations, their industrial counterparts, can take years. Both start by focusing on flavor, which is achieved by adjusting ingredients, proportions, techniques, and cooking times. But while the recipes created for home or restaurant use may also consider ease of preparation and cost of ingredients, once the desired taste is achieved, the work is pretty much done. With formulations, it's just beginning. Now the food technologist has to figure out how to maintain the same flavor and texture over many months or years, and to ensure that no spoilage or bacterial contamination occurs.

This balancing act is what makes the shelves of ingredients in Natick's small "traditional" kitchen—an alcove with a stove, a sink, pots, pans, and ladles off the western side of the industrial-equipment-jammed pilot lab—so jarring. Tins of oregano, thyme, nutmeg, and cinnamon are interspersed with big silver cans of cheddar flakes, banana flakes, and dehydrated peppers. Plastic tubs of Maltrin, a combination of cellulose and guar gum, and carrageenan are mixed in with the flour and sugar. Calcium sulfate, ascorbic acid, and sodium lactate are lined up like bottles of vitamins. Today the Natick Center food scientists are comparing how glucono delta-lactone and pHase, both of which lower the meat's natural pH level, affect the taste, stability, and safety of the sandwich. They won't know the answer for two more months—and then, depending on the results, may have to make more tweaks to the formulation. No wonder this item has been in development for almost twenty years.

LeBlanc and Anderson roll the loaded baking rack of sandwiches across the pilot plant. On our way, we pass oversize Hobart and Blodgett mixers, kettles, combination ovens, conveyors, and compactors. The meat-filled rolls are proofed—allowed to rise for an hour in a humid chamber—and then "baked off" for thirteen minutes in a walk-in industrial oven. (And, yes, there's a handle inside just in case.) After the sandwiches have cooled, we bring them over to the packing area. A young technician, Lauren Pecukonis, holds open small plastic pouches, each labeled with their storage times (T-0, starting time; 2 weeks; 4 weeks) and whether they are a control or one of the two variables. LeBlanc waits until the last minute to cut open a package of oxygen scavengers—there's a small hiss as they awaken and begin to feed on the air around them, then quickly drops them into each bag. She hands the packet to Pecukonis. "Vacuum-seal it! Quickly!" A loud whoosh. "Oops!" Pecukonis looks sheepish. She's accidentally vacuum-sealed shut the vacuum sealer.

The easiest way to understand the importance of this packaging to the food it contains is to imagine skinning yourself. (If the thought is too macabre, I'll allow you to substitute a banana.) The consequences are dire. First, the physical barrier between your insides and the rest of the world is destroyed, causing a big disgusting puddle of blood and guts to leak out. Second, a host of microbial invaders rush in, consuming your vitals and spreading disease. Finally, air, water, light, and temperatures that are either too cold or too hot bring about changes to cells and substances. Let's be frank: you're not long for this world. Similarly, without its wrapper, that chicken fajita entrée or giant soft chocolate chip cookie isn't either. (Although an unstinting hand with the chemical preservatives can do a lot to hold these forces in check.)

The food technologists admit as much. "I'd like to be able to say that formulation is everything," says LeBlanc. "But to be honest, the reason we get the stability we get is the packaging."

The Polymer Film Center of Excellence, run by Jeanne Lucciarini, a neatly dressed blonde in a sweater set, is where designing this vital packaging takes place. The room, which is no larger than forty by sixty feet, is crammed with equipment, including five laboratory-size extruders that, with their long barrels and squat, vertical hoppers, look sort of like giant staplers. The machines melt plastic pellets, called resin, and then push the softened material through a specially cut hole. The Natick Center's equipment produces films, either cast (rolled) or blown, and often in two or more layers simultaneously (the Collin Teach-Line Multilayer Co-Extrusion System can do a whopping nine). These multi-ply wrappings, which may include foil and paper as well, allow rations to last so long, go anywhere, and endure all sorts of physical abuse. Their latest projects, Lucciarini says, focus on nanocomposites, microspheres (which puff up in the film, decreasing the weight and the amount of plastic needed), and biodegradable packaging (the army estimates that each soldier generates eight pounds of waste per day in camp, the bulk of which is plastic and paper).

Once all the sandwiches are sealed into pouches and put into two cardboard containers, we're ready for the penultimate step: a visit to the warehouse that runs along the back of the main building, where the Natick Center operates what amounts to an amusement park for boxes. Here rations are tested for durability and longevity with rides full of the careening, spinning, jostling, and sloshing that children find so inexplicably pleasurable. There is a drop tester, which hauls packed rations up to the height of a hovering helicopter and then lets them free-fall to the ground below. A compression tester squishes packages between two heavy metal plates, sort of like a giant horizontal mammogram. Over in the corner jiggling merrily away sits a vibration table, which simulates the effect of three hundred miles of bad road in a flatbed truck. We deposit the boxes in the environmental chambers, one of which is set to Bangkok (120°F, 90 percent relative humidity [RH]) and the other to Baghdad (120°F, 5–10 percent RH). I step into each. The dry heat is fine; the moist wilts me like boiled lettuce. Our samples will enjoy a four-week vacation before being opened and checked for spoilage and flavor deterioration.

I won't be here to enjoy the results, but the Natick Center has arranged for the next best thing: I'm going to act as an evaluator for some sandwiches prepared eight months ago. "I'm going to have to lower my standards," jokes Sensory Evaluation Coordinator Jill Bates. Usually panelists undergo a rigorous three-month training program before they are let loose on the two thousand consumer-market and one thousand in-house development food items that must be tested every year, which they can then describe with professional terms such as "interfaces," "cell structure," and "flavor migration." Bates hands me a paper plate with half a sandwich, a plastic fork and knife, and a napkin and guides me to one of the dozens of computer stations that line the walls. I sit down, and when prompted by the instructions on the screen, bite, taste, and swallow. Overall, my ratings fall short of positive: The "sausage looks a little congealed," the "smell [is] overwhelming and slightly repellent," although I relent and concede the snack as a whole is "surprisingly tasty!" (I am not, however, the harshest in my panel of tasters: Tester 07788 calls the bread spongy, and Tester 02327 slams the conglomeration of meat, cheese, and bun as "soapy/almost moldy.")

For dessert, a technician has laid out what appear to be several tubes of toothpaste. Tube foods, developed for fighter pilots decades ago, can be hooked up under your oxygen mask and require absolutely no chewing—solids can be so troublesome at 5g! I squirt some into a plastic spoon and taste. They are to real food what a book review is to a book: the simultaneous presentation of an idea—the browned meat and onions, simmered tomato, and a pleasant cheesy top note: easily identifiable as sloppy joe—without all the work of plowing through and assembling everything yourself. The apple pie is just as good, a full-frontal assault of apples with a hint of cinnamon, suspended in a buttery crust. For one wonderful moment, I feel like Violet in *Charlie and the Chocolate Factory.*

★ ★ ★

THE DAY IS DRAWING TO A CLOSE. I've seen dozens of technicians in lab coats. I've seen hundreds of shiny machines. I've been suitably impressed by the long list of food-processing firsts and amused by some of the wackier-seeming inventions. But there's something important missing.

It's the suite of offices off toward the left end of the building, where figures occasionally emerge and disappear, a pair of black doors flapping behind them. I don't ask to be taken in, because what would there be to see, anyway? People hunched over their computers. Someone talking on the phone. A group huddled around a conference table. It wouldn't look like much. But it's there that the real work of steering America's processed-food industry takes place. The labs I've been visiting all day are a smoke screen.

Chapter 3

AMERICAN FOOD SYSTEM, CENTRAL COMMAND, PART TWO

59,422 breakfast sausage patties

98,220 eggs

21,082 packages sliced American cheese

2,451 containers frozen apple juice

13,500 packages julienned French fries

24,159 corn dogs

8,682 frozen burritos

To say the U.S. military buys in bulk is an understatement—the above shopping list is from a single prime vendor contract for facilities near Seattle, Washington, and Hermiston, Oregon, in 2002. The weekly grocery needs of the entire armed forces could pick clean whole regions of their number one agricultural products, leave bare-shelved commissaries across the country, and tie up battalions of baked-goods manufacturers for months. It's essentially one giant mouth munching the American landscape, and, despite commanding deep discounts on its purchases, with $3.8 billion in annual spending in 2011 alone, it is far and away the nation's leading institutional grocery buyer. (In the private sector, the annual expenditures of behemoth food distributor Sysco and monster restaurateur McDonald's exceed those of the Department of Defense.)

These dollars, managed by the Defense Logistics Agency (DLA), the military's purchasing agency, affect the American food industry as might those of any big spender—red carpets and gold-plated customer care, which means conversations between the agency and industry that probably go something like this: "Hello, Commander, any new contracts on the horizon? The crust was a little pale on the breakfast pastry? We'll be right on that, sir. You'd like to add some functional ingredients to the processed cheese spread; what would that entail? You were approached by a tofu factory in Oregon about making a soy ginger noodle entrée? Very exciting, but wouldn't it be easier for you if we just added a soy entrée to our regular line?" These accommodations may orient commercial production to mess halls and combat rations, but it's not the military's prodigious purchasing power that's turned the food industry into G.I. Joe's brainchild.

No, that happens at the Natick Center, which, in pursuing its mission to "actively leverage leading edge technologies to ensure the warfighter is provided the decisive edge in all aspects of combat feeding," has infiltrated practically every packaged food in the land. Of course, many, if not most, of the lab's daily tasks are humdrum—approving new items for the Meal, Ready-to-Eat (MRE) ration, arranging for a small run of prototype plastic pouches with tear notches, and evaluating stainless steel serving pans for the navy are all par for the course. But there's a whole other category of activity—identifying basic and applied science needs, finding and working with partners for these projects, and disseminating the interim and final results—that exerts a disproportionately large influence on the U.S. food system. This exaggerated power comes not from the size of Natick's research budget, which is relatively small, but from the simple fact of having an overarching goal, a long-term plan, and relentless focus—which, come to think of it, may be the three traits in life most important to making things happen.

The middle section of this book documents the center's impact on particular foods or processes, but to get a sense of how the whole operation happens on a day-to-day basis, let's take a look at the goings-on at the main office at 41 Kansas Street in Natick, Massachusetts, between October 1, 2006, and September 30, 2007 (fiscal year 2007 was the most recent year for which I was allowed information about army partnerships during the writing of this book). It's there that Natick Center staff plans conferences, sets up site visits, and produces presentations. It's there that army scientists and technologists collect information about food industry research and offer expertise to academia, companies, and nonprofits. And it's there that requests for proposals (RFPs)—the documents that describe projects for potential vendors—are written, bids reviewed, contracts awarded, and agreements signed.

The first step is a whole lot of listening. During the year, the Combat Feeding Program talks with "warfighters," the official armed forces term for soldiers, about their wants and needs—more sandwiches, pizza, bagels, and wraps; fewer traditional meat and potatoes–type meals. It gets requests from the various services and agencies. For example, the army might complain: Our guys are sweating off fifteen pounds or getting heatstroke in the field kitchens. How about lowering the temps to below inferno level? The navy might implore: Can't you find a way for us to get equipment onto a submarine other than sawing it up deckside? And it gets general direction from the secretary of defense—decrease the soldier's physical and cognitive burden, reduce the logistics environmental footprint, enhance operational efficiency—who, in turn, gets his or her marching orders from the Defense Science Board, the military's quadrennial plans, and presidential science and technology policies.

"The Army solicits the entire community in terms of what needs improvement in combat feeding," explains Gerard "Gerry" Darsch, who was director of the DOD Combat Feeding Directorate from 1994 to 2013. "It could be something very simple. It could be something very complex. And it could be something that requires a lot of high-risk, high-pay-off investment. And not only do we solicit those joint statement-of-need proposals from each service, Natick's team also generates potential joint statements of need in terms of where we think an investment in science and technology can bring new capability to the battlefield. You really have to have a vision in terms of looking over that fifth ridge, if you will, in terms of a potential solution that would affect the shelf life, the quality, minimize logistics, make it more lightweight, cost-effective, and also include the nutrition warfighters need—even the food-service equipment because that's a major part of the program as well."

All of this information is presented twice a year for approval to the Department of Defense Combat Feeding Research and Engineering Board (DOD CFREB). Until the early 1980s, this committee was an outside group organized by the National Academy of Sciences–National Research Council (NAS-NRC) and drawn from academia, industry, and the armed forces—in fact, it dates all the way back to the World War II Committee on Quartermaster Problems. Today it is an internal group composed solely of brass from the army, Marine Corps, navy, air force, and DLA, and chaired by an official from the Office of the Assistant Secretary of Defense for Research and Engineering, a civilian who's also part of the Senior Executive Service, an elite corps of government workers trained to lead, manage, and interpret policy. At each of these meetings, small adjustments are made. "In some cases, we recommend that programs be terminated; in others, that things be accelerated; and in still others, that dollars be shifted," says Darsch. "What we do better than anybody else is we develop a ten-year program that specifically maps out the amount of time, what the end state of each research category needs to be, and a specific transition from basic research into technology demonstration and then through what we refer to as the 'valley of death'— moving to commercialization." At the end of the process, the Combat Feeding Program spits out a detailed set of research and development plans, complete with objectives, tasks, and timetables, for the year.

These projects generally fall into three categories, each of which corresponds to a number in that most shock-and-awe-inspiring of documents, the Defense Budget Justification, the annual tome put together by the armed forces to persuade Congress to continue to fork out their more than half-trillion-dollar allowance. There is 6.1, basic scientific research, which is largely undertaken at universities and in DOD laboratories, of which there are eighty across the country. There is 6.2, applied research, or getting that science to actually do something useful; this happens at universities, DOD labs, nonprofits, and industry partners. And then there is 6.3, figuring out how that something useful can be manufactured; this part of the technology transition process is almost always parceled off to industry. (The Defense Department actually has four more categories, 6.4–6.7, which correspond to manufacturing the item and getting it into the field; these are the favored feeding ground of mammoth military contractors such as Lockheed Martin and Northrop Grumman.)

To carry out all these different kinds of research projects, the army has at its disposal an alphabet soup of joint ventures, some of which receive government funding, and therefore must abide by reporting requirements, and many of which do not—although they receive a host of other supports—and therefore occupy a vast, mysterious landscape about which little is known. These collaborative undertakings are one of the most important mechanisms through which the Natick Center influences the food industry. In fiscal year (FY) 2007, there were 275 such partnerships. There are the Broad Agency Announcements (BAAs), in which institutions and firms compete for basic research and development projects closely defined by the Combat Feeding Program; their benefit to the contractor is primarily financial. There are Small Business Innovation Research (SBIR) awards, which fund businesses with fewer than five hundred employees to seek the answer to technological problems in the hope that this will spur the development of new products. In FY 2007, the Combat Feeding Program had eleven SBIR awards. Many of these were for the development of competing versions of solar-powered refrigerated containers, waste-to-energy converters, and individual beverage chillers; although spending on them was low, these projects may very well influence the consumer market of the future (they are described toward the end of the book). Such straight-up contracts are cursed, however, by the need to comply with government purchasing rules, the Federal Acquisition Regulations (FARs), which require reports on everything from annual revenues and taxes to executive compensation, all laid out in a breezy 1,887-page document.

Then there are the looser arrangements: Patent License Agreements (PLAs), where companies lease military patents for fun and profit; and Educational Partnership Agreements (EPAs), through which the military supports targeted science and technology education for college, high school, elementary school, and even—I kid you not—beauty school students. There are also Memorandum of Agreement (MOA) partnerships, in which the military reimburses a nonprofit educational institution or other government agency for its services; Memorandum of Understanding (MOU) partnerships, in which it does not; and Dual Use Science & Technology (DUST) partnerships, in which both parties contribute funds and share the right to use the end product. For example, as C. Patrick "Pat" Dunne, a retired Natick senior scientist, explains, "Microwave sterilization was really spearheaded by Natick through a dual use science and technology program we initiated with industry and academia. . . . Down the road we're going to produce that in the military, and it's going to become big in the commercial sector, too."

And finally there arc the crown jewels of the Defense Department research program: Cooperative Research and Development Agreements (CRADAs) and Other Transactions (OTs). All those complaints businesses have about working with the government—burdensome and intrusive administrative regulations, book-length proposals, demanding socioeconomic requirements, and heavy-handed managerial oversight? Gone. And the rewards? Staff time, services, laboratory facilities, equipment, and materials are theirs for the taking. The significant difference between CRADAs and OTs is that partners cannot receive payment for their participation in CRADAs but they can in OTs, as long as they don't "profit" from the arrangement.

Still, that doesn't explain why major food conglomerates such as Campbell Soup Company, ConAgra, Dr Pepper Snapple Group, Frito-Lay/PepsiCo, General Mills, Graphic Packaging, Hormel Foods, Kraft Foods Group, Mars Inc., Michael Foods, Procter & Gamble, Rexam PLC, SoPakCo, and Unilever are lining up to enter into cooperative agreements with the Combat Feeding Program. In FY 2007, Natick's food division was involved in eighteen separate CRADAs, amounting to a finger in every promising new technology from mini vacuum cleaners for pathogens and membrane-based juice concentrators to high-pressure processing for produce and nutrient-fortified candy and bakery items; they even had an agreement—resulting in a lawsuit*—to commercialize the HooAH! energy bar. Big corporations get involved in CRADAs because they expect something in return: a piece of the vision Natick has for the future of food. As Evangelos of the Combat Feeding Directorate pointed out, industry research tends to be at science's margins and focused on consumer appeal rather than at the forefront of innovation. When companies work with the army's subsistence department, whether they receive an exclusive patent or a head start on a breakthrough processing or packaging technology, they get the chance to dominate the market when new products based on it come shooting out of the pipeline.

★ ★ ★

ACCORDING TO LAWMAKERS, making sure government-funded research and development gets used in new commercial products is exactly what federal agencies should be doing. It's called technology transfer and when it happens, it's like a Disney movie for grown-ups: businesses pop up like flowers, employees break into song at their desks, bankers drape rainbows across the sky, and tax collectors tap-dance down the street.

The policy dates back to just after World War II, when the head of the wartime Office of Scientific Research and Development (OSRD), Vannevar Bush, persuaded the government to invest in public science, primarily through universities, to maintain U.S. technological superiority for military readiness and as a deterrent to enemy hostilities. These activities were managed by civilian-controlled laboratories working in close cooperation with the armed forces, and later other branches of the government. The U.S. Army Natick Soldier Research, Development and

---

* The army had entered into an agreement with California-based D'Andrea Brothers LLC to commercialize the snacks, but then began purchasing them, using the same name, from another vendor. D'Andrea Brothers sued for breach of contract. In February 2013, the U.S. Court of Federal Claims found in favor of the plaintiff but did not award damages.

Engineering Center is one of these laboratories. (There are about seven hundred more, some big, some small, and each with a different focus.) At times this arrangement stimulated the development of new products, but because most of the intellectual property from these projects accrued to the federal government, technology transfer, at least as measured by first-generation impacts, was sporadic at best.

By the late 1970s and early 1980s, after a decade of stagflation, a recession, and a contraction in the manufacturing sector, Americans looked west and were alarmed to see Japan, their mild-mannered protégé, in ascendance, perhaps even poised to dominate the global economy. So they did what any quick-witted competitor does under the circumstances: I'll have what he's having—in this case, a national industrial policy. In Japan that meant targeting high-risk but high-return industries, such as cameras, cars, and semiconductors, and then playing a combined coach-cheerleader-moneylender role to ensure that they prospered. The United States wasn't able to stomach quite so much government intervention, although one might argue that financing the majority of the country's R&D is precisely that. Instead legislators passed a series of laws intended to encourage the federal labs and industry to get intimate.

The romance between government and industry officially began in 1980 with the Stevenson-Wydler Technology Innovation Act, which made it an explicit part of a lab's mission to transfer the technology it developed to state and local governments and the private sector. A few months later, Congress passed and President Carter signed into law the Bayh-Dole Act, allowing academia, industry, and nonprofits to own the intellectual property—usually a discovery or invention—that resulted from a government contract. (At the time, there were twenty-eight thousand government-owned patents gathering dust on U.S. Patent and Trademark Office shelves.) In 1982 lawmakers created the SBIR program to encourage the labs to park some projects with small high-tech companies. But business was still diffident—all those killjoy bidding and reporting requirements. Who needed the headache? In 1986 Bayh-Dole was amended so that the government could enter into a new kind of relationship, the CRADA, that accommodated the private sector's desire to do things friends-with-benefits style (that is, fewer rules, more rewards). Various other tweaks were made, but perhaps the most significant was DOD's ultimate concession, the OT, enabled by statutory provision in 1994, which allowed the industrial sector to do practically everything it ever dreamed of—even get paid for work on which it would keep the patents. Business and government got cozier and cozier, presumably spawning more technology transfer than ever before.*

Which is a good thing, right?

Maybe.

The federal government finances about one-third of all science and technology research and development in the United States, which in FY 2007 was about $370 billion (an investment two to three times that of our closest competitor, China). Of that, although expenditures are broken down about evenly among the three categories—basic, applied, and development—it is by far the most important sponsor of basic research at 59 percent, and relatively less important for development at 18 percent. In our sample year, defense spending on research and development was $82 billion, 60 percent of the federal total. The category percentages flip, however, when compared with the government's as a whole: DOD accounts for only 6 percent of federal outlays for basic science and 18 percent of those for applied, but a whopping 90 percent for development (which makes complete sense when you think of the colossal machines made by companies like Boeing).

The truth is that within the rarified sphere of science and technology,

---

* In a 2012 interview, Cynthia Gonsalves, the former director of the DOD Office of Technology Transition, who wrote the CRADA policy for the services, said, "There wasn't a lot of information [on the impacts of CRADAs] if you look at T2 [technology transfer] and what it was supposed to accomplish, because there was no funding for tracking information, and [we] hadn't established what criteria to judge agreements by." This is seconded by two researchers at the National Defense University in "Public-Private Cooperation in the Department of Defense: A Framework for Analysis and Recommendations for Action," a report issued that same year: "There is no single process, assessment framework, or standardized approach for establishing a [DOD] CRADA or assessing its effectiveness."

the U.S. economy has a lot more in common with the socialism of the People's Republic of China than it does with free-market economics. The fact that the government (and, within it, the Defense Department) is pretty much the only game in town—especially when it comes to basic science—means that research projects are put together with it in mind. You can study anything you want, but if you want to make a living at it—and most academics do—then it needs to be something that attracts funding. And that often means working on one of the many areas deemed essential to the armed forces. The savvy junior scientist knows that if he or she wants to get ahead, the easiest way is to work on a research topic— and handily there are quite a few—related to warcraft.

Then there's the overwhelming strength of DOD's own planning apparatus. The yearly priorities set by trade and professional associations such as the American Association for the Advancement of Science, the American Chemical Society, and the National Environmental Health Association have about as much teeth as that annual rite of self-flagellation, the New Year's resolution, when compared with the regular bottom-up and top-down information gathering, concerted analysis, extremely long time frames (five, ten, twenty-five years), global perspective, and deep pockets (so forgiving when you make a mistake) of the strategy and goal setting of the U.S. military. From this come the precepts that are used to define a welter of specific science and technology projects, which are dispersed each year into the eagerly waving hands of academia, industry, nonprofits, and other government entities like strings of beads at a Mardi Gras parade.

The net effect of all this is that the Defense Department has a disproportionate influence on the direction of many industries, even if basic and applied science is only about a quarter of its research budget. As noted in a 2012 report by the House Committee on Armed Services, "Basic research is especially important in this process of innovation, as it often leads to new areas of knowledge, such as new materials, sensors, nanotechnology, and data extraction, etc., that in turn lead to new areas for development and commercial opportunity. . . . The predominance of basic research for DOD is carried out by the universities. That has in turn led to a trend of increased activities related to commercialization of technologies on university campuses to more quickly translate research into industrial products."[1] (That influence often expands once you get beyond the first generation of impacts—papers, patents, products—but is harder to trace.)

DOD's grip on the business sector is just as tight. "Sustaining Critical Sectors of the U.S. Defense Industrial Base," a 2011 think tank report, poses the question, "Does the DIB [defense industrial base][2] function like a normal free market in which the forces of supply and demand dictate efficiency, innovation, and pricing?" and answers with a resounding no. The Defense Department sees absolutely nothing wrong with this. Close ties and careful guidance are needed to ensure that it has contractors in the areas it needs, when it needs them. In fact, the goal for the twenty-first century is to strengthen its puppet master role. According to the House Committee on Armed Services, "[One of the] challenges to ensuring that the industrial base is positioned to support the needs of the nation in the 21st century . . . [is] the lack of a comprehensive DOD strategy for managing and maintaining an industrial base."[3]

So what? you might ask. Who cares as long as the result is a wellspring of nifty gadgets and cool new products for us consumers?

There's the rub. A now-venerable 1986 UN report observes: "The development of military technologies has an effect on the direction of technological change that goes beyond the simple diversion of resources from civilian innovation. A set of factors—basic principles, technological preferences, performance requirements, nature of the demand—have a strong effect on the kind of technologies developed by the military, in ways that have reduced efficiency, slowed down civilian applications and distorted the overall direction of technical change."

We do have a national industrial policy, one that has run roughshod over the free market of ideas, force-feeding federal—largely DOD—research goals into the hungry craws of craven scientists. This model does not let the best science and technology appear and grow organically in response to a multitude of societal factors—in the case of food, the concerns of farmers, consumers, public health officials, and even the food industry itself—but rather they are chosen and directed along a preordained agenda set to achieve military dominance on the world stage.

★ ★ ★

THE REAL WORK OF THE NATICK CENTER is nothing like the gee-whiz, mad-scientist laboratory tour, and that's exactly the way the army likes it. Because if we noticed what they were really doing, we might object—or at least question what it is we get out of the deal. The effect of their guiding basic and applied food-science research means that discoveries are oriented, first and foremost, to the military. And the effect of their bestowing huge conglomerates with free or low-cost patents and the latest food processes and technology means that the food these companies produce is a close cousin to the army ration.

In this ordinary office suite west of Boston, for reasons that have nothing to do with your health and well-being, your tastes and preferences, or your pocketbook, a group of men and women chose the techniques that are used to manufacture practically everything you now eat—and are choosing everything you will eat in the future—from high-pressure processing, which flattens bacteria so you can pig out on guacamole stored for months at room temperature during Monday night football, to individual beverage heaters, so you can gulp hot coffee brewed in its serving container as you barrel down the highway at 80 mph during your morning commute. (Late again.) In fact, if we noticed what they were doing, we might be horrified to realize we've created a perfect system for training compliant warriors. The fact that we've been tearing open granola bars (a military invention) since we were toddlers makes it seem normal for soldiers street-fighting in Kandahar to bite into a highly compressed emergency ration bar composed of cheap grains, sugar, and protein supplements. *Bon appétit,* America!

The Combat Feeding Program's budget is really rather small—$44 million in FY 2007, a high for the decade, but still just about six ten-thousandths of military research funding overall, with the portion spent on basic and applied research a scant $5 million. To put that in context, let's go into your yard. See that tree, that maple over there, the one that blesses you with dozens of yard bags' worth of organic debris every fall? Let your eye follow the stately trunk, the spreading branches, the clusters of twigs. See that leaf fluttering in the wind all the way at the top? That's the Combat Feeding Program—a tiny piece of an enormous whole. For you to fully understand the impact of the military on your life, take what you learn in this book and multiply by thousands. It's that big. It's so big, it's unimaginable, and if we were to try to erase it, we might end up erasing modern existence itself.

Chapter 4

A ROMP THROUGH THE EARLY HISTORY OF COMBAT RATIONS

T he combat ration—as opposed to the garrison ration eaten in camps—didn't just appear out of nowhere. Like most things, it has a past, and, as with most things, its past informs its present. So let's take a look at the very first foods carried by soldiers on the march or in armed conflict. Which, as it so happens, means going back to before the dawn of human history.

★ ★ ★

IF TO SOMEONE WITH A HAMMER, everything looks like a nail, then what does everything look like to someone with a spear? You got it: prey. The exact moment when mankind (and I do mean mankind, because women have almost always sat out this particular social institution) first lifted hand against his brethren is lost to the murky swamps of prehistory, but at some point, an early hominid gazed at the flint-headed stick in his hand and thought, "I could go track a great mastodon for a couple days, and, with a lot of luck, stab it to death, drag it six miles back to the cave, and then have dinner for me and the missus, or I could just use this on Grok, take the meat he's got already piled up around his grotto, and call it a night." This was unlikely to have been a long, drawn-out decision.

After that, interpersonal violence appeared with depressing regularity. In locations as far-flung as eastern Africa, southern Europe, the Canadian Arctic, and the American Southwest, early humans got busy bludgeoning, impaling, and puncturing one another. Motives? Acquisition of a few days' supply of raw woolly mammoth and a heap of grubby tubers. A cave with morning sun and running water. A hot helpmate. Personal animosity. And—there's no delicate way to put this—a neighbor with some mighty succulent-looking gluteals. Cutting, banging, chopping, and peeling marks on skeletal remains as well as ancient myoglobin-laden (a protein unique to human muscles) *Homo sapiens* poop have made it amply clear that our forebears were not averse to the occasional feast on friend, foe, or frenemy.

For the minimally minded, the Paleolithic (2.5 million–10,000 BC) and Mesolithic (10,000–5000 BC) eras offered an idyllic lifestyle: short bursts of food production (guys: hunting; gals: gathering) punctuated by long periods of lounging about doing nothing; easy-to-maintain living spaces; the stimulation of always going to new places and seeing new things. But eventually (warning: crackpot theory ahead!), the ladies became dissatisfied. They wanted something more. They wanted a place to park the offspring other than a hip. Relief from the frustration of returning to their secret berry bramble or nut-tree stand only to find that someone else had already been there. A place where they could indulge that irrepressible impulse to fluff dried grass and arrange rocks in conversation areas. And, most important, a husband who wasn't always out with the guys on excursions that often seemed more about the thrill of the chase than a serious search for steak, delicious as it was when it materialized. (Not to mention the occasional encounter with comely females from other tribes.)

In other words, they wanted real estate.

Thus began a nagging campaign that probably lasted for centuries. "Move? Not again! We just moved last week. Break down camp. Set up camp. Break down camp. Set up camp. Then spend half the day looking for a couple hummingbird eggs and a handful of fruit. And all that with an unweaned two-year-old hanging from my teat. I just want to settle down. If we stayed in one place, I'd have more energy. I could help skin and cook the day's catch. And I wouldn't be snoring every time you wanted to renew our conjugal bonds." Nothing worked. Until one day she discovered in a dank corner of the current cave a forgotten gourd into which she'd chewed and spat some wild grains to help Paleobaby transition to solid foods. It's strangely frothy. She sips. Eureka! Alcohol has been discovered. From then on, she finds persuading her significant other strangely easy. "Honey, if we had a permanent dwelling, for argument's sake let's call it a house, I'd plant a bunch of grains and make that new beverage you really, really like." In no time at all, she found herself ensconced in a cute little cottage surrounded by fields. (That man invented agriculture so he could keep a buzz on is a bona fide theory proposed by several archaeologists, including Patrick McGovern of the University of Pennsylvania and Brian Hayden at Simon Fraser University in Canada. Should you need further proof, look no further than ancient Sumer, where more than 40 percent of crops were grown to produce beer.)

Of course, just like today, not all guys were ready to give up their inner wildmen. For these, there was another option, something halfway between hunting and farming: herding. Following around a bunch of sheep and goats all day may not have been quite as macho as tracking wild animals and waving penetrating projectiles, but they still got to roam the plain, sleep under the stars, sport matted beards and layers of dirt, and dine al fresco on charred meat and milk. By contrast, their sedentary brothers had settled into a life of grueling manual labor fueled by a monotonous diet of porridge, mush, and legumes and made only just bearable by copious quantities of this newfangled fermented grain beverage. On the plus side of the farmer's ledger: he had food stores (which necessitated the invention of food preservation, mostly by drying but also, when sodium chloride was readily available, in seawater or mineral deposits, by salting), buildings, land, and due to an increased birthrate, nubiles. On the minus side: all these things looked mighty attractive to the herders, who, with their rough-and-tumble ways and well-practiced knife skills, frequently descended en masse and spirited the pluses away.

The tension between these two lifestyle choices and the bloodshed it engendered became one of the epic narratives of the Neolithic age (8000–2000 BC). In ancient Sumer, Dumuzid the shepherd and Enkimdu the farmer vie for the favors of Inana, goddess of love, fertility, and war. The other tale, which is probably a later version of the Sumerian one, is much better known: that of farmer Cain and shepherd Abel. The first sibling rivalry—which is tastier, my veggies or your lamb chop?—ends in the first murder, a fact which should only be of surprise to the childless. After many millennia, these archetypes still echo (just think of the vitriol between vegetarians and carnivores) and spawned two opposing styles of warfare, as well as the rations that fueled them: the orderly agriculturists who ate carbs gussied up with a bit of protein and sauce and the wild mountain people who subsisted on meat and milk.

Like the turtle of Aesop's fable, the farmers plodded on, bound and determined to make something of themselves. They bred beasts of burden. Assembled sticks into rudimentary plows. Dug ditches to bring river water to their plants. Eventually their nose-to-the-grindstone approach paid off, and they began generating extra food, which meant not everyone had to spend his day from sunup to sundown in the fields. Gilgamesh decided to dedicate himself to pottery; Anu to metalwork; Ur-Nammu, to bossing everyone around, especially in the all-important areas of water rights and land disputes. And Tizkar, Lugalkitun, and Untash-Gal, armed to the teeth with spears, clubs, and bows, to looking and acting very scary (even easier once these were topped by sleek bronze weapon heads instead of rocks). With the birth of cities came the need for organized violence—to defend them, expand them, and police them.

The goon squads had arrived.

And they needed to be fed. This was easy enough on home turf, when soldiers were generally supplied with meals by the government or given provisions—but what about on campaigns, when men were expected to fend for themselves, an act militaries euphemistically call foraging, but we civilians know as raping, pillaging, and plundering? Sure, the first few times it may have been a head rush to enter a new village and have the townspeople prostrate themselves before you, begging for their lives and proffering their worldly goods. But the routine got tired fast. Leaders quickly figured out that portable edibles allowed recruits to spend more time on the job and less time starving, miserable, and harassing the locals for chickens and turnips.

Herewith a quick tour of some of the world's major military empires and their combat rations with emphasis on those that have most influenced the West.

★ ★ ★

THE FIRST STANDING ARMIES APPEARED with one of the first two civilizations (as measured by the blossoming of its flower, bureaucracy), that of the Sumerians (3500–2200 BC), who inhabited the fertile plains between the Tigris and Euphrates Rivers from the middle of the fourth millennium. In addition to cuneiform, base 60 math, and sacred prostitution, the Sumerians, who spent two thousand years in ceaseless warfare among their fourteen or so city-states, invented some really kick-ass weaponry and military techniques. However, their rations know-how remained primitive, probably for the simple fact that most of their excursions were so close that soldiers could go home for lunch and still have time to return for a full afternoon of socket-axing and sickle-swording. (The first war ever recorded in detail, on the Stele of Vultures, was between Lagash and Umma, only eighteen miles apart.) When they brought something along to munch while doing victory laps in their souped-up chariots, it might have been beer (of which they were inordinately fond), a few barley cakes, and green onions. (Apparently, halitosis was not a big concern during classical antiquity.)

The ancient Egyptians (3200–1000 BC), who kept up with their (distant) neighbors the Sumerians in almost everything—agriculture based on flooding and irrigation, food surpluses allowing division of labor, cities, and government—were behind when it came to the arts of war. It wasn't their fault. It's easy to get complacent when you're cut off from the rest of humanity by an ocean (to the north), large deserts (east and west), and a mammoth river with several churning waterfalls (south), discouraging to even the most foolhardy mariners. For over a millennium, the

Egyptians did their own thing—his and hers extreme makeovers, dragging immense boulders up ramps, and oversharing on that breakthrough communications technology, paper—until they were invaded by the Hyksos, a seminomadic tribe from the east.

So much for isolationism. It took them more than a century, but with the help of some copycat weaponry—the chariot, composite bow, sword, and penetrating axe—endless training, and the adrenalizing effect of hate, the Egyptians rallied and ran the rubes out of town. Then, what with a military infrastructure already on pharaoh's payroll, they took it one step further and went expansionist themselves, reaching Nubia to the south, and to the east, Palestine, Babylon, Assyria, and the Hittites. By 1500 BC or so, they'd rolled up so much new territory, the sons of the Nile were holding down some four hundred thousand square miles at once. To manage the flow of food and fodder to this vast network of garrisons and camps, the Egyptians invented a new profession, the quartermaster, who, using small naval vessels and oxen, kept the men in beer, bread, onions, and dried and/or salted fish—this last so important that soldiers received an allotment every three months as wages.

In fact, these piscatory provisions (also used by the Assyrians) were a rations revolution: lightweight, imperishable, and highly nutritious. Sure, you could munch bread during combat or stop and make porridge while on a long trek, but by far the most efficient thing you can eat in terms of replenishing the body's supply of amino acids, the building blocks of cells, is some form of dried or compressed meat (or, somewhat less completely, dairy). It may well have been this portable protein that enabled the Egyptians to range so far and wide, amassing distant territory. And every great empire since has been powered by at least one reliable preserved protein that could be carried and eaten as is while marching, doing surveillance, or even during combat.

The ancient Greeks (750–323 BC) were nothing if not paramount mythmakers. Democracy? Just one tiny city-state out of more than fifteen hundred was truly democratic, and that privilege was only extended to free male landowners. Elegant architecture and sculpture? Turns out the temples and statues were painted a garish red, blue, and yellow. Their military prowess and exploits have dominated the Western canon largely because they bothered to write them down (from them we inherited our perhaps misguided notions of glory and heroism), but in point of fact the Hellenic armies—despite centuries of endemic warfare over the hard-scrabble lands of their hilly little peninsula—were mostly small bands of amateurs armed only with sword, spear, and shield (they did invent an important military formation, the phalanx). Their rations, which were carried by individual hoplites (soldiers) for a maximum of three days' march, were similarly rudimentary: several pounds of grain, sour wine, the ubiquitous onion, and, for their portable protein, pressed rotted milk from mountain-grazed goats, also known as cheese.

But there was one exception to this dilettante approach, a place where career commandos thrived: the militocracy Sparta, which led the allied Greek city-states to victory over Persia in 479 BC. Tough-guy training began at birth when weak babies were euthanized, and the ones who survived were given really rotten childhoods, consisting of early maternal separation, random beatings, and food deprivation. But when future warriors arrived to adulthood, their early privation was more than compensated for by their privileged positions as Sparta's only citizens and landholders. After age twenty-one, esprit de corps was maintained with compulsory communal dining in local mess halls, meals that always began with the same none-too-subtle appetizer, a black broth consisting of vinegar, pig's blood, and porcine body parts. (This soup was the butt of many classical-era jokes.) The rest of the dishes came from mandatory contributions—mostly grain, wine, and cheese—from the men's farms, which were worked by helots, a slave class, whose disproportionate numbers—nine to one—kept their masters on their toes.

Later, Philip II of Macedon finally unified Greece (359–336 BC) and implemented several reforms that foot soldiers undoubtedly rue to this day, including prohibiting the accompaniment of wives, consorts, and prostitutes (they ate too much food and slowed down the march) and compelling each man to carry his own rations and equipment, an innovation that burdened the Greek recruit with eighty-pound packs, thirty pounds of which were two weeks' worth of grain. (Modern American soldiers carry even more; their rucksacks, water purifiers, rations, and arms weigh a full one hundred pounds.)

It should please Italophiles to hear that the Roman Republic and Empire (509 BC–AD 476) were built on pork, specifically prosciutto (air-cured ham), bacon, and sausage. Each foot soldier, or legionnaire, marched with a string of sausage, a hunk of Parmesan or other hard cheese, and a bit of *lardo* for cooking in his bag. Other ingredients for an on-the-move meal were *garum*, fermented fish sauce (soldiers actually got a cut-rate version), and hardtack, a crispy twice-baked flour-and-water concoction, ancestor to the cracker. These staples could travel to the ends of the extensive empire—in its heyday, Rome controlled territory from the British Isles to North Africa and from Armenia to Egypt—without spoiling. Well fed, well trained, well equipped, and super buff (their centurions kept them in top form by parading them around the countryside wearing seventy-pound packs), Roman combat soldiers easily dominated the ancient world for a millennium.

Recruits ate well during campaigns—in a thousand years, nary a complaint was made about the chow—but in the garrison, they feasted. In fact, the life of the sedentary warrior pretty much revolved around food. At his disposal were vast military bodegas stocked with grain, *carnaria* (racks of meat), hard cheese, dried fruit, and condiments; terrains for growing vegetables and raising livestock; requisitions or purchases of food from the surrounding countryside; and, most important, regular correspondence with loved ones to badger them into sending care packages. He baked bread. He hunted hares. He demanded asparagus, cabbage, wine, and fine olive oil, and, as did one soldier in the below letter to a friend, got snippy when these did not materialize.

> Rustius Barbarus to Pompeius, greetings. First of all I pray that you are in good health. Why do you write me such a nasty letter? Why do you think I am so thoughtless? If you did not send me the green vegetables so quickly, must I immediately forget your friendship? I'm not like that, or thoughtless either. I think of you, not as a pal, but as a twin brother, the same flesh and blood. It's a

term I give you quite often in my letters, but you think of me in a different light. I have received bunches of cabbages and one cheese. I have sent you by Arrianus, the trooper, a box, inside which is one cake and a *denarius* (?) wrapped in a small cloth. Please buy me a *matium* of salt and send it to me without delay, because I want to bake some bread.[1]

Undergirding this military might was an agricultural productivity the world had never seen before or since—at least not until the twentieth century. The Romans considered working the land to be the noblest of all occupations; their nascent empire was built by citizen-farmer-soldiers as only the landed could belong to the army. (Later, as Rome conquered new enemies and acquired their territory, a vast system of latifundia, or slave-worked plantations, arose; their large tracts of monocrops were a precursor to our factory farms.) And what animal best complemented these verdant fields and orchards? Not the high-maintenance chicken or cow, delicious though their eggs, milk, and—at the end of their working lives—cadavers were. No, what the ancient agronomist most appreciated was the easygoing pig, which lives on scraps and forage, which drops litters of eight to ten twice a year, and which achieves a squealing full-size corpulence in a mere six months. Perhaps most important to its central role in the early Italian diet, preserving these tons of pork was no longer prohibitively expensive. The Roman Empire, which controlled the world salt trade, distributed an allotment of the crucial mineral to soldiers as part of their wages and, when necessary, artificially lowered its price in the marketplace. A whole new world of *salumeria* was born— and traveled with the legionnaires to every corner of the empire.

Being on a Viking longship would have been a lot like Beer Pong Night at Phi Sigma Kappa: a few dozen grunting, sweaty dudes packed into a small, none-too-tidy space; free-flowing keggage (contrary to legend, this was water, not ale); and a wholehearted belief in the supremacy of force over reason. Starting in the late eighth century until the last decades of the eleventh, the vessels, which were designed for speed and maneuverability, departed from the Scandinavian coast and set out for sea towns in France and the British Isles. On board, the men subsisted on a dispiriting diet of barley mush and butter, enlivened by the occasional slab of dried halibut or cod. Although fish were abundant and easily dried in the northern climate, the Norse were primarily an agricultural people; early warriors, all landowners, left their farms entrusted to the hands of slaves and local peasants. The repast was not prepared shipside but at numerous pit stops along the way, some at stone towers previously stocked with dried fish and meat, cereals, cheese, butter, and beer. The raids themselves were brutal and short—the Vikings were skilled at hand-to-hand fighting, and when all else failed unleashed their secret weapon, berserkers: wildmen high on reindeer piss who were fearless in battle. Although they lacked an overarching political structure and military coordination, the Norsemen dominated northern Europe for several centuries through sheer savagery.

The Mongols (AD 1206–94) were the herders' last hurrah—and they validated the idea that the right rations make all the difference. They assembled, albeit briefly, the largest land empire ever known. (The Huns, who knocked on Rome's door, then stomped through and wrecked all the furniture, were lightweights by comparison.) Exceedingly mobile, self-sufficient, and vicious, they were in many ways the forerunners to today's special ops. The Mongols were consummate horsemen (the horse, until it was replaced by the combustion engine, was for several millennia the ultimate in battle transport); they literally lived in the saddle and rode for days on end simply by rotating mounts from the string that ran behind them. They were impervious to pain, cold, and discomfort—from an early age they slept on even freezing ground without blankets. But most important, their rations—protein-rich powdered milk that they turned into shakes in a saddlebag and strips of homemade jerky cured under the saddle with horse's sweat and the weight of the rider—turned out to be the perfect warrior food (portable, convenient, lightweight, and nourishing) and may have been central to their military might. (When these ran out, the Mongols had an infallible emergency ration: hot blood drunk straight from a vein in their horse's neck.)

After the Mongol Empire's peak—it stretched from Siberia and

Southeast Asia and eastern Europe to the Middle East and its armies killed an estimated fifteen to thirty million people—the nomadic lifestyle, with its tents and ruminants, went out of style, absorbed into the great teeming cities with their grain-based economies. Echoes remain in ancient antipathies expressed as food prejudices: the Chinese distaste for milk and dairy products, staples of the Mongols who conquered them; the Muslim and Jewish—the Semites were the original wanderers—prohibition against swine (animals unable to digest grass, resistant to herding, and not built for trekking), which was an instinctive sneer at the livestock of the enemy; and even our own fetishization of the juicy steak, a hidden reference to our barbarian past (the Angles, from whom the Anglo-Saxons descended, were cattle herders). The Mongol legacy also persists in the powdered milk and jerky that still stock soldiers' rucksacks today.

If there was ever an argument against eating an all-vegetarian diet it's the Aztec civilization (AD 1427–1519). By the Paleolithic era, all large native herbivores in the Mesoamerican basin had been hunted into extinction, so when agriculture began there it was not accompanied by the simultaneous domestication of livestock found in other cradles of civilization. Undaunted, the early Mexicans cobbled together a barely adequate diet of nixtamalized maize (treated with an acid-neutralizing solution that frees niacin), beans, and chilies enriched with an occasional zap of protein from iguanas, lake scum, and insects. The only two kinds of livestock were reserved for nobles: turkeys and Chihuahuas, which, given their diminutive size and extreme boniness, can only be considered a measure of their misery. Battle rations weren't much meatier than commoner fare, consisting of maize three ways; beans; pumpkin, chia, and amaranth seeds; and the ubiquitous hot peppers. It was thus perhaps inevitable that the protein-hungry Aztecs' gaze alighted on the one large mammal that continued to grace the Valley of Mexico: man.

What ensued was one of the most bizarre and bloodthirsty warrior cultures on the planet—and, please, if you have a weak stomach, skip this section entirely—which kept the elites (nobles, priests, and soldiers) well nourished and the masses (peasants) weak and docile. Between 1427 and

1519, the Aztecs, an alliance among three city-states, bellies growl-
ing after repeated maize crop failures, were led first by Itzcoatl and
then by Moctezuma (and later his descendants) to conquer adjoining
territories westward to the Pacific, eastward to the Atlantic, and as far
south as Guatemala. But unlike other military imperialists, the Meso-
americans had little interest in the traditional spoils of war—property,
goods, power—and except for collecting regular tributes, most of them
edible, allowed their conquests to return to business as usual, with ruling
structures intact. This was because they had already obtained the natural resource they most wanted: a fresh harvest of enemy soldiers.

If the everyday Aztec warrior diet lacked the soul-satisfying experience of masticating a hunk of thermally processed mammal muscle,
feast days more than made up for it. War captives, after being plumped
up in special holding cells, were marched up the temple steps; at the top
a priest sliced open their chests with an obsidian knife, plunged his hand
in, and held the still beating heart up to the sun. Once the religious cer-
emony was out of the way, the serious eating began. The body was tumbled to the base of the building, where it was quickly turned into prime
cuts by attendants. The skull went on a trophy rack; a thigh was reserved
for Moctezuma; the flayed skin was used for a grotesque game of trick
or treat in which young warriors bedecked in fresh person-hide went
door-to-door asking for food; the rest of the limbs went home with the
victim's captor so he could invite over all his best buds for a heaping bowl
of human stew (the warrior himself was not allowed to eat his own captives). It's estimated that, over its century reign, the Cannibal Empire
devoured more than one million men, women, and children.*

★ ★ ★

EATING AND WAR HAVE BEEN INTERTWINED since the very beginning. Animals fight over food; so do we. And while it's easy to forget in a world

---

* The extent to which the Aztecs practiced cannibalism and why are still being debated
  by anthropologists. The "ecological" theory described here was proposed by Michael
  Harner and is not universally accepted.

where there are tempting tidbits at every turn, just ingesting enough calories not to starve to death used to be an all-day proposition. There were two distinct post–Paleolithic era strategies: herders and farmers, which eventually melded, as did the dietary styles associated with them. That the recurring conflicts over our most important resource, or the land used to produce it, were fierce and bloody should startle no one. Nature is cruel and capricious: Weather is erratic. Disasters strike. Populations increase. The obvious solution to this insecurity was to amass more subsistence, or the means to it. To support this never-ending quest, cultures evolved foods for warriors that were light and rugged for easy transport, were dried or salted for long storage, and provided optimal nourishment, often a protein. If that sounds familiar, it should. These are exactly the same qualities—with a few tweaks—that modern-day armies seek in developing and perfecting combat rations.

Chapter 5

DISRUPTIVE INNOVATION: THE TIN CAN

F or thousands of years, armies had been content to rely on folk knowledge to prepare the foods they took into battle. Beginning in the late eighteenth and continuing through the mid-nineteenth century, the Industrial Revolution, which introduced machines and expanded markets, turned that relationship on its head. In a role reversal that continues to this day, the military, relying on its hand-maidens science and technology, began to muck about in the kitchen, inventing and helping to promulgate new ways to preserve, store, and transport food.

★ ★ ★

IF YOU THINK WE LIVE IN A TIME OF TURMOIL, you should have been around three centuries ago. Punch-drunk on ideas like freedom and equality, radicals and rabble-rousers overthrew monarchs right and left and hounded the common man into participating in representative democracy. Emboldened by a move away from theism, scientists dared to declare that the universe did not, in fact, revolve around us and, further-more, was controlled by preposterous ideas such as gravity and the laws of motion. Pushed off the land by enclosures, which put shared grazing grounds into private ownership, and driven into cities by the lure of earning a pittance for piecework, the European population became increasingly urban. But amid all this transformative hubbub, warcraft—and rations—stagnated.

Peek in the rucksack of the French or American Revolutionary soldier and what would you find? Almost exactly what you'd seen in that of the Roman legionnaire almost two thousand years earlier: flour, legumes, hardtack, and a chunk of bacon. This made perfect sense given that no new food-preservation method had been invented since man, at wit's end with the excess corn, cabbages, and critters from his farming success, embraced drying, salting, smoking, and fermenting.

Sort of a why-fix-it-if-it-ain't-broke approach.

And then it did break—during the French Revolutionary Wars, when the *citoyens*, with the zealotry of all new converts, decided to "persuade" the rest of Europe (modern-day Britain, Austria, Belgium, Germany, Italy, Luxembourg, the Netherlands, Portugal, Russia, Spain, Switzerland, plus Egypt thrown in for good measure) as to the validity of their views. A ginormous army of 1,500,000 men aged eighteen through twenty-five was raised—the first universal conscription in modern history—and all that testosterone needed fuel. General Napoleon Bonaparte, a baby-faced dictator-in-training, implemented a two-pronged feeding strategy while on campaign: a backbone of staples, schlepped in by boat or beast, and, for everything else, a standing order to go wild in the towns and countryside (fine in summer and fall, not so much in winter and spring). This made logistics speedier and more flexible than the traditional supply chain, but had a few—rather gaping—holes. One was that the troops might be MIA when a vital battle rolled around because they were off plundering the countryside. Another is that they might end up weak and ravenous because there was nary a foie gras nor a *pain de campagne* to be found.

In response to these field-feeding foul-ups, the logistics nightmare of arranging *bœuf bourguignon* for 1.5 million, and the yawping ghost of starvation left over from the Revolution, the French government issued a challenge in 1795, backed by the equivalent of one year's salary. Were there any would-be food technologists around who could come up with a "composition of a work on the art of preserving, by the best possible means, every kind of alimentary substance"? This foresight has ever since been attributed to Napoleon, who, like all megalomaniacs, had a knack for suctioning up every achievement in the vicinity, even those that weren't his. The fact is that in the early 1790s, the Little Corporal would have been far too preoccupied engineering his meteoric rise through the French military, sweeping the Paris streets of royalist riff-raff, and courting the notorious French cougar and heartless harlot Joséphine to have spent time with a bunch of midlevel bureaucrats at the Department of Agriculture talking about food-preservation techniques. Of course, the story might have been different had he known its importance would far eclipse that of his other accomplishments, including the concept of a unified Europe and the Napoleonic Code (excellent if you happen to be on good terms with the judge, less so if your only hope was appealing to the nonexistent jury).

The government's call for help was answered by a bad-boy celebrity chef turned candy man. By the time he was in his twenties, Nicolas Appert, an innkeeper's son with no formal education, had clawed his way up the kitchen ranks to cook for high society—dukes, duchesses, princes, and princesses. In his thirties, already jaded from the glamorous life, he opened a confectionery shop, an experience that would serve him well—better perhaps than training in physics, chemistry, and biology—in his quest for applied-science glory. He observed the magical effect of low, steady heat on taste, texture, and—when the glass container was tightly sealed immediately afterward—spoilage. The bain-marie, a metal container set into another metal container full of boiling water, is indispensable equipment for producing dairy-based sauces, creams, and custards; melting chocolate; and making flavored syrups. It maintains a constant temperature because boiling water, as it's at the exact point where liquid turns to vapor, can only boil faster, but not hotter. Appert would also have noted that fruit prepared in syrup, jams and jellies, or alcohol and stored in stoppered glass containers could last a long time without going bad. (These delicacies also relied on sugar as a preservative and an antimicrobial.) For more than ten years, the entrepreneur conducted painstaking experiments with vegetables, meats, dairy, soups, and stews in sealed bottles cooked in a water bath.

Of course, like any smart businessperson, Appert had his eye not only on the onetime prize but also on the possibility of a lucrative ongoing contract as a supplier to the French military. In 1803 he made his move, delivering his most delectable goods—soup, boiled beef in gravy, and peas and beans—for field-testing to the navy. Three months passed before he heard back; they'd passed with flying colors. Then, silence. A couple of years later, he delivered more samples. Again, they passed with flying colors, and again nothing came of it. (As anyone with government-contracting experience can attest, the modern-day process hasn't sped up much.) Six years went by; Appert expanded his "spring, summer and fall in a bottle" business—so-called because people could eat "fresh" produce all year round—to a bustling forty employees; he delivered yet another round of samples. Finally, in 1809 he received a formal response: everything was satisfactory, except for the beef broth, which was deemed "weak." He was invited in for the big presentation, and a month later Napoleon's minister of the interior awarded him the 12,000 francs—on the condition that he relinquish ownership. Appert, poor sap, did.

The invention did have one flaw: the bottle. Glass was fine and dandy for middle-class families seeking to add out-of-season produce to the table, but impractical for naval or land expeditions (unless for mission-critical supplies such as spirits and wine). Luckily, at about the same time across the Channel, Peter Durand was inventing—and smartly patenting— the tin can. The first can factory, which opened in 1813, was not a high-volume operation; at full tilt, a skilled artisan crafted six to ten containers a day that were then filled with cooked food and simmered for up to six hours apiece. At this low output and (presumably) high price, the only early adopters were the British army and the Royal Navy, which ordered gargantuan cans of stew and soup for long journeys or expeditions. By the American Civil War, however, the ability to manufacture small cans cheaply and efficiently and the resulting reduction in cooking time turned the product from luxury good or emergency ration to everyday soldier fare, although the only tinned food bought in any quantity by the Union army was condensed milk for officers' messes and army hospitals. (Enlisted men had to buy their own from sutlers, the peddlers who trailed behind the army with sundries and snacks.)

Today, the inventor of the fifth major food-preservation method is immortalized by the technique that bears his name: appertization. That's right, appertization. What do you mean you've never heard of it? It's the process of heating a liquid or solid food to a steady, high temperature to kill harmful microorganisms. But that's pasteurization, you say? The sad reality is that fifty years after Appert's discovery, along came Louis Pasteur, draped in degrees, who claimed all the credit. To be fair, Pasteur actually understood the underlying scientific principles—that many illnesses are caused by microorganisms and that these can be eliminated or at least drastically reduced by heat treatment—while Appert simply figured out that the technique worked. But still. You'd think that the man who'd dedicated his life to discovering the single idea that has most changed the face of food in the last two hundred years would have earned more than the occasional impassioned paean from food nerds like me.

★ ★ ★

A CENTURY AFTER APPERT DISCOVERED CANNING, its industrial use had grown by leaps and bounds, especially in Australia and the United Kingdom, where there were strong markets for condensed milk and tinned beef. In the United States, Gail Borden's 1856 invention of canned condensed milk had caught on quickly, but the Chicago meatpackers, whose refrigerated carcass business was booming along with the railroads, saw no reason to diversify. It would take a mammoth order for canned beef from the U.S Army, a very public crisis, and an even more public exoneration to pave the way for public acceptance of this newest way to preserve animal protein.

Between latitudes 23.4378° N and 23.4378° S, in the geographic region known as the tropics, the weather is very pleasant for three months a year, conveniently coinciding with northern postholiday ennui and the frigid temperatures that wither the desire for outdoor adventures, and steamier than the sixth circle of hell the rest of the time. It was here that the United States danced her 1898 debutante cotillion—partner: Spain—as an international military badass, in the process relieving him of several torrid little islands (first Cuba, then Puerto Rico, the Philippines, and Guam). It should have been a cinch, except for one thing: when planning the very first invasion of the Spanish-American War, the army had forgotten to take into account that Cuba is very, very hot.

The problem was the meat ration, which, for the first time during a war, was supplied chilled or in cans rather than on the hoof. Refrigerated beef carcasses had been sold commercially since the 1870s, so it was natural that the armed forces would adopt the simpler, cheaper way to prepare and ship red meat. But the inclusion of canned animal protein was a novelty. The three big Chicago meatpackers—Armour & Company, Swift & Company, and Morris & Company—that had dominated the industry since the Civil War hadn't taken up "beef canning . . . on a large scale"[1] until 1879: not coincidentally until just after the army ordered that heat-sterilized meat be part of the travel ration. (At the same time, the navy unceremoniously incorporated it into sailor fare, to the tune of some five hundred thousand pounds a year.) Thus, when the next full-fledged military conflict, the Spanish-American War, erupted, there was a radical changeover—from traditional fresh or salt-preserved to the first modern processed food.

By early 1898 the meatpackers were on a bovine bender, buying up cattle for rations to send to Puerto Rico and Cuba. In addition to the thousands of tons of "refrigerated beef," which were transported by special railway cars and ships but sometimes experienced what are known in the trade as "temperature abuses," short or long periods of time out of the cold, they cooked up hundreds of thousands of pounds of canned beef and delivered wagonloads to Tampa, Florida. Where they sat on the sunny dock. And then were shipped in sweltering holds. And then were left on the blazing beach for days on end. When the soldiers finally received these rations, they were shockingly ungrateful. Some reactions:

"It made myself and my comrades gag."

"The sight of it turned men's stomachs."

"Our company dog would not eat it."

"The smell of this tinned meat was so vile it could not be opened without opening the car window."

"When partaken of at evening mess it caused violent cramps in the stomach during the night."[2]

"At the best it was tasteless; at the worst it was nauseating. . . . It at once became putrid and smelt so that we had to dispose of it for fear of its creating disease. I think we threw it overboard."[3] (This last comment was made by future president Theodore Roosevelt.)

When American troops sit at a chow hall table or open a can of government-issued rations after a long day of bayoneting, Gatling-gunning, and defilading on behalf of their fellow countrymen, they expect the kind of solid nourishment befitting a world-class power, not something that elicits the gag reflex. Although acknowledged belatedly—a complaint was registered after the war ended by Major General Nelson Miles in a tell-all to the *Kansas City Star*—the outrage at the camp in Santiago de Cuba sent shock waves through the military command hierarchy and ultimately reverberated through the halls of Congress. Matters were made much worse by the fact that many soldiers had already been weakened by typhoid fever in the stateside base camps and besieged by yellow fever once they'd landed. Two thousand, four hundred, and eighty-five enlisted men died of illness during the Spanish-American War—almost eight times the 385 men who died in combat.

But that was only the first act of the Cuban gristle crisis. In late 1898, a federal investigation was initiated by President William McKinley; the Dodge Commission met 109 times, heard testimony from 495 witnesses, and issued an eight-volume report running thousands of pages. Laboratory testing was done, but even the ornery United States Department of Agriculture (USDA) chemist Harvey Wiley, a fervid antipreservatives proselytizer, could find no traces of the alleged boric acid, sulfites, salicylic acid, or benzoic acid (then common meat preservatives) and reluctantly affirmed that the canned meat was unadulterated. Careers were ruined: General Miles, the commanding officer who'd lobbed the first verbal grenade—"embalmed beef!"—was rebuked for not addressing his concerns through proper channels. General Charles P. Eagan, head of the Commissary Department, was court-martialed and convicted for his intemperate reply. "He lies in his throat, he lies in his heart, he lies in every hair of his head and every pore of his body, he lies willfully, deliberately, intentionally and maliciously."[4] And other careers were launched: Teddy Roosevelt, whose Cuban exploits made and broke the mold for manly men, rode the brouhaha all the way to the White House, first as vice president and then as president after McKinley was assassinated. In fact, the episode's repercussions are felt to this day: in 1906 Roosevelt pushed through Congress the first Pure Food and Drug Act; government, academia, and the food industry began to conduct real research on how to kill the microorganisms that live in food; and the army completely overhauled its systems for procurement and feeding of troops in the field. The chastised Lieutenant General Miles, on the other hand, eventually retreated to the sidelines, his name forever sullied by his "ruthless, unjust attack on the Commissary General of the Army," as it's described in his Arlington National Cemetery biographical sketch.

But was he, in fact, wrong?

★ ★ ★

BY ALL ACCOUNTS, Lieutenant General Miles was not a nice man—vain, overweening, and prone to shooting his mouth off. His long military career was as often marked by internal skirmishes as it was by external ones. However, in the case of the stinky steaks, he may well have been speaking the truth—an unpleasant one that neither the military nor the meatpackers wanted to hear, and especially did not want bandied about in the press, as it would have disrupted the move to cheaper and more efficient ways to serve meat to soldiers and, ultimately, civilian consumers. The hearings were cast as a meticulous investigation into the incident followed by an impartial assignment of responsibility; in fact, both the process and the findings supported the interests of the military and industry. The commission overemphasized some of the accusations and sidestepped others. It made authoritative declarations of findings when none were warranted.

Let's review.

First, what exactly were Miles's charges against the U.S. Army Commissary Department and the federal government? Dr. W. H. Daly, a surgeon on his staff (Daly committed suicide a couple of years after the scandal), concerned for his patients, inspected—but didn't test—several shipments of refrigerated beef, and found it to have "an odor similar to that of a dead human body after being injected with preservatives, and it tasted when first cooked like decomposed boric acid."[5] Based on this, the good doctor believed that the beef had been treated with chemicals, a charge championed by Miles, who declared it to be a "secret process of preserving beef."[6] (It's notable that in the report Dr. Daly remarked on the taste of boric acid, an impression the army triumphantly dismissed because boric acid has no taste or odor.) The army duly tested other meat shipped to Puerto Rico and found it to be free of adulteration. On the other hand, only passing attention was paid to proving that spoilage had not occurred en route, although it was stated that "the testimony, with some exceptions, showed that the refrigerated beef issued was pure, sound, and wholesome."[7]

With regard to the canned beef, the army made the same argument as to its integrity—a fact that Miles had not disputed—while avoiding a prolonged discussion of its deterioration, about which it conceded: "There is no doubt that when issued to soldiers in Cuba and Porto [sic] Rico, where it was exposed to the heat, and where they did not have the proper means of treating the cans, as directed on the labels, and could not properly cook it, the meat was unpalatable, especially to those suffering from malaria, or convalescent. . . . In a tropical climate, carried on the march, exposed to heat, the meat so changes in appearance as to become repulsive."[8] It was this point that General Miles had made, about both the refrigerated and the canned beef, and which, with its righteous indignation about the accusation of chemical preservation, the War

Department did not refute but buried under the voluminous evidence it presented to prove that no tampering, intentional or not, had transpired.

Little did any of these actors realize that four hundred miles north in Cambridge, Massachusetts, key evidence that could have been used by the defense had already been discovered. In 1895 a lowly assistant to a Massachusetts Institute of Technology (MIT) professor, a young man named Samuel Prescott—who would later become a dean and founding president of the Institute of Food Technologists (IFT)—was tossed the thoroughly unprestigious assignment of helping the local William Underwood Company figure out why their canned clams kept exploding. Prescott and Underwood's work on the bivalves, as well as other canned seafood and vegetables, was published in 1896, and became the first studies on an essential food-processing concept, thermal death times—the times and temperatures at which bacteria and their spores are killed. This finding, however, would not yet have reached the ears of the army Commissary Department or the Chicago meatpackers who, like the rest of the world, had only just accepted the theory that sickness was caused by germs, tiny organisms (in fact, thermal death times would not become a foundational precept of the canning industry for another quarter century). Since then, our understanding of and ability to control the microorganisms that spoil and poison food, not to mention the forces that cause its physical and chemical deterioration, have exploded. Looking back at the "embalmed beef" scandal with more than a century's worth of microbiology, bacteriology, and food chemistry at our fingertips, we can determine with a lot more precision what exactly happened. But first, let's take a brief foray into the ways food can go bad.

★ ★ ★

THE ESSENTIAL FACT OF OUR EDIBLES is that they are dead—lifeless plant (although fresh fruits and vegetables do continue to respire) and animal tissue already half embarked on the inevitable journey to decay. (Thus the disconcerting similarities between the laying in of food stocks and the mortuary sciences: pretty much every traditional way of storing sustenance—drying, salting, sugaring, smoking, and burying—has been practiced on the human corpse.) Some of the changes are the result of simple physics and chemistry, driven by randomness or gradients. Others are wrought by our invisible cohabiters, the fungi and bacteria that populate our insides and outsides, our homes and gardens, soil, water, and air. Food preservation's most important task is to defeat these—anthropocentrically speaking—dark forces, which, for the first time, can invade plant and animal tissue and items made from them without having to contend with the formidable defenses of living cells. It must slow or halt the spoilers, which are all over anything expired and which can make a mess of things in as short as a few hours for fresh shellfish to years for dried grains and nuts. And it must destroy the poisoners, for which we are the ideal—or at least one—habitat and whose residency can cause anything from a grumbly tummy to an agonizing death.

Some of food's problems are simple senescence, sometimes set in motion by electromagnetic waves emanating from the sun. Visible light, which occupies a relatively narrow range of wavelengths, is the sun's most abundant kind of radiation, and drowns the earth. Conveniently, the energy level of its photons is just right for powering terrestrial chemistry; certain wavelengths of visible or lower-energy UV light make an electron jump to outer orbitals in the atoms of many of the ninety—or hundred—or so naturally occurring elements (scientists disagree on their exact number), making them more reactive. Thus, in food, sun or other light can cause some molecules to decompose, others to glom on to new ones, some to rearrange themselves, and still others to become charged.

An example of one of these changes is lipid oxidation, a complex set of chemical reactions in which two or more molecules do an electron shuffle, in the process creating a new set of molecules. (An oxidant is a molecule that gains electrons from another molecule; a reducer donates them.) When this happens to the fat in stored food, it goes through a chain reaction, producing free radicals (molecules with one or more looking-for-trouble unpaired electrons) that combine with neighboring molecules to cause off flavors, color changes, and nutritional losses.

Anything with fat can be susceptible: vegetable oil, butter, meat, dairy, nuts, whole grains, and, of course, fried and snack foods.

Temperature has a similar effect on edibles, although its impact is more generalized and occurs much more often than that of light. Heat from the air enters the food through convection, in which the agitated warmer molecules adjacent to the food pass it some of their energy, in the process becoming cooler and heavier. These cooled molecules are then replaced with warmer ones, which do the same thing, until the temperature of the food and the air are at equilibrium. The food itself heats up through conduction, in which the agitated molecules pass some of their energy to adjacent ones, but without changing position. The molecules in the now-hotter food have more energy, setting off more chemical and enzymatic reactions; these double for every 18°F increase at room-temperature range.

One of the most important of these is the Maillard reaction, or non-enzymatic browning (as opposed to the enzyme-generated discoloration that happens naturally in fruits and vegetables), which occurs when part of an amino acid that has electrons to donate and part of a sugar that can accept electrons combine and then rearrange themselves to form a number of new, highly reactive compounds. These compounds produce a variety of different flavors, colors, and aromas, many of them desirable, for example, the savory taste of cooked meat and the golden crust of bread, and others not, such as darkened packaged pastries, musty boxes of milk, brown dehydrated fruits, and warmed-over-tasting canned meat.

Unlike most of us, food can legitimately blame the majority of its problems on someone else. The minute an organism dies, things go downhill fast. The initial set of changes are internal, and have to do with the continuing activity of enzymes, the uncontrolled release of intracellular fluid, and the halting or breakdown of cellular structures. All others have to do with the invasion of saprophytes, aka death eaters, which are eager for their turn using matter and energy in the food chain, and microparasites caught in between hosts. In edibles, there are two main categories of microbes, fungi (yeasts and molds) and bacteria, which further break down into two classes, spoilage and pathogens.

Although humans can get ill from fungi, it is rarely from ingesting them—at least in the developed world. More often, it's the airborne spores that cause an allergic reaction or out-of-control inflammatory responses (think sick buildings coated with black mold), or that gruesome condition known as mycosis, in which the little buggers sprout on the skin, in the airways, and even in the eyeballs of a *Homo sapiens* host—almost always one who is immunocompromised. In the less fortunate nations (that is, most of them), there's a laundry list of fungi that cause disease through ingestion, almost always by growing on and producing toxins in staple cereal crops (wheat, rice, corn) in the field or during storage. In the United States, however, for the most part, the only mycotoxin of any great concern is aflatoxin, which is found in peanuts and corn (its levels are regulated by the federal government). Aflatoxin is an extremely potent carcinogen; Iraq even weaponized it in the 1990s, possibly for use against the Kurds, though there's no evidence it was ever utilized.

As a rule of thumb, fungi rush in where bacteria fear to tread: low moisture—or rather a related concept called water activity—low temperatures, high acidity, and salty and sugary environments. They come in two varieties: yeasts, which are small, one-celled organisms that can quickly form large colonies, and molds, which are large multicellular strands that are technically a single organism. Some species of both have been our handmaidens in the biotechnological processing of food for thousands of years. The jolly yeasts lighten beer, wine, and bread, consuming sugars and producing ethanol and carbon dioxide. The molds are a more saturnine lot. When they're working for us, they add piquant and earthy tastes to cheese—for example, the reverse eponymous *Penicillium roqueforti* and *Penicillium camemberti*—and umami to soy products. But when they're not, they turn everything they touch ghoulish: colored green, blue, gray, and white and coated with a revolting fuzz. Most spoilage from fungi is in perishable foods, but their spores can be heat-resistant, so if conditions are right, they may occasionally germinate in preserved foods.

You'd think that olfactory red flags—eau de diaper, wet socks, dirty dishrag, and skunk, along with "unspecified bad odors"—would be a clear sign of food that can make you sick. But, in fact, most spoilage bacteria, the beasties that produce the stink, are innocuous. Because they evolved to consume dead plant or animal matter, they tolerate low temperatures (your refrigerator's 35°F–38°F is fine) but languish when the mercury really spikes. In fact, if they could, they'd give us a wide berth. To storm Citadel You, they'd need to survive a dousing in stomach acid (pH 1–2, also good for tanning leather and sterilizing pools); elude the death squads of intestinal immune cells; and withstand an enervating 98.6°F, none of which they're equipped to do. The stench is from their digestive process, which turns amino acids into amines, including the evocatively named cadaverine, putrescine, and spermidine. (As repulsive as they are, only one, histamine, has been linked to serious negative health effects for people who have allergies to it or who eat certain kinds of improperly stored fish.) In your refrigerator ecosystem, the dominant type is probably *Pseudomonas,* species of which are responsible for decorating meats with green slime, spoiling milk, and turning leftover moo goo gai pan fetid. Another class of grocery gremlins belongs to the *Lactobacillus* (LAB) family, which defile meat, milk, and bakery products with acerbity, ooze, and stench. Other LAB branches produce fermented products such as cheese, salami, and sauerkraut—very niftily, when a healthy batch of LABs dominates the food surface, it protects against the growth of colonizers.

The term *pathogen,* disease-causing, which came into use only in the mid-1800s, is rather egocentric, as if the whole purpose of some bacteria was to ruin your day. The truth is most are just going about their business, which, as is the case for most living things, revolves tiresomely around consumption. That a colony is homesteading on that pile of cafeteria mashed potatoes or that coffee-shop banana cream pie, and happens, when you scarf down your portion, to be given an all-expenses-paid trip to your small intestine, may simply be a case of wrong place, wrong time—even for them. In fact, for some bacteria, we're bad news from start to finish: their encounter with our considerable defenses (see above) leaves the place littered with small, dead bodies; with luck, a few hapless spores or a modest reservoir of poison escapes. Others, the noninvasive pathogens, are able to duck the gastrointestinal bodyguards, but would be just as happy to inhabit your garden or your compost heap as your food or your stomach (one of the hallmarks of bacteria is flexibility—they have multiple ways to metabolize nutrients and generate energy). And then there are a few, the invasive pathogens, who truly are mad for us.

Noninvasive pathogens are like those supercilious outdoorsy types who are always saying there's no such thing as bad weather, just inappropriate clothing. They come prepared—for anything: extreme temperatures, nutrient scarcity, environmental stresses, and immune responses. They get their bearings quickly, and before you can set down your gear, they have mounted a base camp and are scouring the woods to rustle up dinner. Their habitats—or lifestyles, as microbiologists coyly call them— can include soil, dust, water, silage (composty stuff), vegetation, insects, animals, food-production facilities, food, and you. In certain environments, they produce toxins that can be unpleasant or even deadly to humans. But again, there's no need to take it personally: toxins may just be a defense mechanism to disable competitors in the host or other environments. And if things get really dire, they've got a Plan B: little packets of genetic material like seeds that can easily outwait just about anything, from Noah's flood to the Roman Empire—molecular biologists have found viable forty-million-year-old bacterial spores.

The noninvasive pathogens are no gourmets. Like children, seniors, and the vast majority of Americans, they like their comfort food— starches, gravies, filled pastries, meat loaf—which is why they thrive in food-service environments more given to substance than style: buffets, cafeterias, and other institutional settings. Because they are everywhere, it's just a matter of waiting for the right circumstances—say, a nutritious batch of chicken à la king after several hours on an inadequately heated steam table—before they overrun the place. Not that you'll know. Per standard pathogen modus operandi, invasions are done on the down low.

A couple of the more common noninvasive pathogens are *Bacillus cereus,* sometimes called "fried rice syndrome"—it's mad for carbs—and *Clostridium perfringens,* a protein hound who's a regular guest at picnics, schools, and prisons and is one of the most ubiquitous in the environment, equally happy in soil, decaying plant matter, the intestinal tracts of humans and other vertebrates, and insects. Both *B. cereus* and *C. perfringens* are spore-formers, so food may arrive already impregnated with its own unhappy ending—for *C. perfringens,* high-heat cooking even benefits it by promoting germination and killing off competing organisms. A final common noninvasive pathogen, although not a spore-former, is *Staphylococcus aureas,* a resident of the nasal cavities, skin, and sores of infected humans that is also found in soil, water, and air.

By contrast, the invasive pathogens are incorrigible homebodies, luxuriating in indoor temperatures and regular meals. For the so-called microparasites, we—and our farmyard friends, the cows, the pigs, and the chickens—are the cat's meow. Their idea of a good time is to loll, warm and cozy ($98.6°F$ is ideal, although they're also willing to be fruitful and multiply at room temperature), on the tropical beach of our small intestines, letting the amino acids and sugars wash gently over them. While they're waiting for their dream host to appear, they're willing to hang out in your burger, your spinach, or your raw milk. But since this isn't their optimal environment, to do so, they may sacrifice their offspring or enter a suspended state known as viable but nonculturable (VBNC)—they won't grow unless resuscitated. Other strategies for survival in inhospitable secondary habitats include the formation of biofilms, which may explain outbreaks that have been traced to produce.

That's not to say that invasive pathogens are pacific. To invade the promised land, they come as geared-up as a USAF special op. For starters, they're stealthy (as are most pathogens), giving no warning—no noxious odors, no slimy textures, no unpleasant tastes—as to their presence in food. In the stomach, they often become temporarily acid-tolerant. In the small intestine, they bind to and disrupt immunological command centers. And, once established, colonies can turn downright mean, ousting other occupants from preferred perches and monkeying around with the body's natural defenses, such as the protective mucus layer, by releasing toxins. These have a second life as a clever travel strategy. Some of the excreted substances or the infection itself makes you feel very, very sick, triggering a release of bodily effluvia (though, luckily for them, usually not sick enough to kill the host). Greetings, family and friends!

Most cases of food poisoning come from a barnyard trio that spend their lives in a snug circle moving from host to host. *Campylobacter jejuni* populates the intestinal tract of most livestock, especially chickens, but can survive in raw milk, untreated water, and undercooked meat. At ambient temperature, however, it dies quickly, and in food it's easily eliminated by heating, drying, freezing, acidic conditions, and disinfectants. *Escherichia coli* is the world champion of diarrhea, especially among U.S. travelers and children in less-developed nations, of whom 380,000 die annually from dehydration related to the illness. It lives in warm-blooded animals and birds, as well as dung-dirtied food and water. The most common variety is quite mild, but the much more toxic subgroup *E. coli* O157:H7, which first showed up in ground beef and beef products, can be more serious and on rare occasion may cause death. *Salmonella* is the most common cause of bacterial food-borne illness; like the other invasive pathogens, its primary habitat is the guts of domestic and wild animals, both birds and mammals—that includes us—from which it infects eggs, poultry, beef, pork, processed meats, and dairy products. *Salmonella* is handily dispatched with heat, so is not a problem in traditionally processed foods.

Three pathogens should always be treated with the utmost respect, so despite the fact that they belong to both the invasive and noninvasive groups, they get their own special category: cold-blooded killers. Their commonality is a deadly one: a refusal to limit themselves to the gastrointestinal system. (*E. coli* O157:H7 also belongs to this Most Wanted list; it secretes a toxin that after it has breached the intestinal wall enters the bloodstream and damages tiny blood vessels; most victims survive, but a few die of liver failure.) *Listeria monocytogenes* is an oddball among the food-borne pathogens in that it is very cold-hardy, which means that stowing infected raw and soft cheeses, ice cream, sushi, deli meat, and hot dogs in the refrigerator does nothing to halt the proliferation of the bacteria. (In nature it is found in soil, water, vegetation, sewage, and silage.) Like the microparasites, it creates infections. However, once in the gut, the bacteria can cross the intestinal wall to enter the bloodstream, from which they slip into liver or spleen macrophages, white blood cells that engulf foreign matter, a sort of immunological wolf in sheep's clothing. In healthy hosts, these are sussed out and zapped, but in immunocompromised ones, they can then penetrate other organs, including the central nervous system and the placenta of pregnant women, where they may cause brain problems or miscarriage. Another assassin comes from the deep blue sea. Cousins *Vibrio parahaemolyticus*, the more innocuous one, and *Vibrio vulnificus* are both denizens of raw and undercooked fish and shellfish. *V. vulnificus*, if it enters the blood, can cause septic shock and death. The microbe is fragile, requiring a saline environment, and it is easily destroyed by acid, freezing, cooking, and common disinfectants—this is little comfort for raw bar aficionados, however, unless you're willing to turn your clams on the half shell into lemon-marinated ceviche.

There is one bacterium so fearsome it makes food engineers quake in their rubber-soled, fluid-impermeable shoes: *Clostridium botulinum*. The noninvasive pathogen is the most difficult to eradicate of all the "bad bugs." It forms spores at high heat that can persist after processing, thrives in low-oxygen conditions such as cans, and produces a deadly neurotoxin with a high fatality rate. *Clostridria* are all around us in soil and on plants. In food, they usually ride in on an innocuous vegetable proudly "put up" by a home canner: mild asparagus, green beans, corn, or peppers. These low-acid foods offer ideal conditions for germination. (*C. botulinum* can't sprout below 4.6 pH. Accordingly, the Food and Drug Administration [FDA] and the USDA have different regulations for canned low-acid, acidified, and acid foods.) To preserve low-acid foods safely, industry uses a "botulinum cook," 250°F for at least three minutes, a heat unachievable at home without a pressure cooker. If the endospore germinates and grows, the bacteria produce a toxin that, after it's eaten, passes through the intestinal walls and into the central nervous system, where it disables the axons that transmit signals, leading to muscle paralysis and, frequently, death.

★ ★ ★

NOW THAT YOU HAVE A WHIRLWIND TOUR of modern food microbiology under your belt, let's turn our attention back to the scandal of the fetid fillets. Let's start with the refrigerated meat, presuming that there were some temperature violations during transport, at its final destination, or both. The beef was shipped in carcasses, which means that almost all microbial colonies would have been on the surface of the meat; this lets off the hook food-preservation enemy number one, botulism, which only occurs with anaerobic environments. The sides of beef could easily have been contaminated with microparasites during slaughter, which inhabit the intestines of warm-blooded animals and have a nasty habit of spilling out during dismemberment. But they are heat labile and not spore-formers, so the army's presumably thorough cooking before serving would have destroyed them. The same goes for any fungi or spoilage bacteria that might have hitched a ride from the carcasses' point of embarkation or during the journey, although the latter could very likely have left an unpleasant calling card, the biogenic amines that are the product of their metabolism. The fact that the surgeon who started the whole mess claimed to smell boric acid and other adulterants suggests this, as amines are not inactivated in cooking and can cause nausea and diarrhea. If the refrigerated carcasses were causing serious illnesses, by process of elimination, these were likely imparted in the camp through handling of the meat before serving. In fact, even in the twenty-first century United States, the vast majority of food-borne illnesses are bestowed by the human touch; a full 58 percent of cases are from noroviruses. (Viruses are not a problem in stored or preserved food as very few live long outside a host.)

Now to the canned protein; was it the culprit? According to the Dodge Commission report, the beef had first been cooked, then canned in two- and six-pound tins and sterilized for two to three hours at 215°F–225°F. Given that the seals hadn't ruptured—and there were no reports that they had—this is more than sufficient to kill all live bacteria and spores. (Even though most modern processors eliminate botulinum spores with higher heat for a shorter time period, a cook time of about an hour at 215°F is also sufficient.) This serious overcooking would have also destroyed any fungi, spoilage bacteria, or other pathogens in the cans, as it would the taste of the meat, producing unpleasant nonenzymatic browning. Add to that some lipid oxidation brought on by storage in high heat, as well as assorted other unpalatable but nondangerous chemical deterioration, and—voilà: canned food you wouldn't give your dog.

The "embalmed beef" scandal may have shaped American food safety law and practice, but the truth is that if any Spanish-American War soldiers died of gastrointestinal illnesses in Cuba and Puerto Rico, they most likely contracted them there—not from the rations, although these were in some cases spoiled and in others terribly decayed. Did General Miles really deserve to go to the grave shrouded in ignominy from the dustup? He spoke the simple truth of the senses, a truth that the science of the time could not explain, and unwittingly became the fall guy for the missteps of the military and the food industry in their mad rush to modernize American meat eating.

Chapter 6

WORLD WAR II, THE SUBSISTENCE LAB, AND ITS MERRY BAND OF INSIDERS

I magine that you're preparing an intimate dinner for 12 when you suddenly receive word that instead you'll be feeding 385 people and they'll be at your doorstep in a matter of hours. This situation is a little like the one faced by the Quartermaster Corps during World War II, when, over the course of four years, the U.S. Armed Forces had to ramp up production to provide three square meals a day for from four hundred thousand to almost twelve million recruits. This enormous task descended on a tiny Chicago laboratory formed almost as an afterthought and headed by a cavalry officer with no professional food-service experience, a B.A. in chemistry, and unproven leadership ability. Over the duration of the war, the organization was transformed. The soldier, valiantly working with almost no resources, enlisted the help of food companies, big and small, and, on a later project, even brought in a couple of university experts to do nutritional and acceptance testing.

But it wasn't enough. The rations rusted and tasted bad. So the army assigned control of the lab to a consummate businessman who was famous for slashing through red tape and inspiring employees; he expanded the internal research program and set up an external one, under the watchful eye of one of the country's leading food-science experts.

But it still wasn't enough. Canned milk jelled; dried potatoes hardened; fats went rancid; preserved meat, eggs, vegetables, and fruits browned. By the end of the war, "to cover all fields of interest to the Armed Forces, but also to stabilize the whole research program on military subsistence,"[1] a massive outside science and technology program was begun under a second food scientist coordinating almost five hundred projects spread among university, company, and government labs throughout the country. What had once been a small, fly-by-the-seat-of-your-pants operation had become a professionalized research juggernaut and the driving force behind the development of processed foods—then and now.

★ ★ ★

COLONEL ROHLAND ISKER HAD ALWAYS LIKED TO COOK, a passion he'd deepened in the Pacific, where he was stationed in the Philippines from 1919 to 1923, acquiring both a taste for Asian cuisine and, as a token of appreciation for his services, a gift watch from Japan's Prince Nashimoto. But as a lieutenant in the U.S. Cavalry, the mounted forces even then being made obsolete by armored tanks and trucks, he didn't have an opportunity to do so professionally until, at the age of forty-four, he was enrolled in the army's Subsistence School in Chicago, which taught personnel how to purchase and prepare edibles to feed troops. Two years later, in 1939, he was finally assigned a food-related tour of duty: making sure the electricity, water, heat, and refrigeration were running at the Chicago Depot of the Quartermaster Corps, the army branch that provides soldiers with food, water, and other supplies. As a postscript, Isker was also told to manage the newly created Subsistence Research Laboratory because its founders, Colonels Wilbur McReynolds and Paul Logan, had been summarily reassigned to the Washington, D.C., office.

The lab couldn't have been sleepier: three staff, including the director; a couple of donated pots and pans; and a special projects budget of $750. It had been formed as restitution to McReynolds and Logan, instructors at the Subsistence School who suddenly found themselves jobless when it moved to Philadelphia in 1936. The idea of a lab was part of their impassioned plea for employment: "The Subsistence School . . . had investigated many promising food developments for the army, but its work, in the main, had not been experimental. . . . A research laboratory, however, with teaching omitted from its program, might be expected to observe a completely new function."[2] In addition to his nonexistent staff, equipment, and funds, Isker inherited two production-ready projects: a deliberately unpalatable emergency chocolate bar developed after years of fiddling by Logan and then perfected by Hershey, and the C (for combat) ration, a gray and mushy meat stew in a can that was the personal inspiration of McReynolds. Said the colonel of his invention, "It was a radical departure from the previous rations, and, of course, soldiers would rather have steak and gravy and potatoes. But the C-ration eliminated the need for transportation space on ships going abroad and that was what sold it."[3] It was not exactly a plum post.

That all changed on September 1, 1939, when a notorious brush-mustached thug invaded Poland, and France and Great Britain, galvanized by the attack on their ally, declared war. The United States, dolefully watching the unrest outside its window to the east and to the west, went on high alert. On September 16, 1940, Congress enacted a draft, requiring all men between the ages of twenty-one and thirty-five to register for military service; that year, the army, navy, and Marines added almost two hundred thousand new recruits. Wartime preparations were also under way at the Subsistence Research Laboratory: its special projects budget was increased—by $50 to a total of $800. Isker was undaunted. Under the eye of Logan in the Washington Quartermaster Corps office, he scoured the country for consumer products that could be added as they were, or with minimal changes, to the rations. Sniffing war contracts on the horizon, twenty industry representatives a day were visiting the lab by the end of 1940.

The Germans had taken the world by storm not only with military prowess but also by scientific supremacy. Borrowing a page from their book, the United States, whose armed forces enrollment had now tripled to more than 1.6 million, elevated the role of science in its war strategy, in 1941 establishing the Office of Scientific Research and Development

(OSRD) to fund research into weapons, explosives, communications, equipment, and soldier support, among other things, and appointing a former MIT vice president, Vannevar Bush, to head it. The Subsistence Research Laboratory also grew, albeit modestly, to a staff of twenty-two and developed multiple labs, including a chemistry lab, a vitamin lab, a kitchen, and a dining room. Still, research and development dollars were short, and Colonel Isker continued to make up the difference by working with "civilians and scientists who were drafted from large food companies," according to Research and Development Associates, the organization he founded after the war. The day-to-day work of the Subsistence Research Laboratory was mostly standardization: developing set menus, writing instruction manuals, figuring out nutritional content, testing items, and creating detailed specifications for the manufacture of countless products and packaging, according to Kellen Backer, who wrote his Ph.D. thesis on the topic.[4]

Isker also began work on the first Subsistence Laboratory item to rely on university researchers in its development, a lightweight emergency ration for those deployed in planes, helicopters, motorcycles, and tanks. Complaints had been received about the C ration, specifically that its six twelve-ounce cans were awkward, heavy, and at times downright dangerous for soldiers to carry. MIT offered an updated recipe for the pemmican-in-a-can (the mixture of dried meat, fat, and berries used by Native Americans) that had been used in World War I, which would have reduced the size and weight, but struck out. Field tests done by Ancel Keys at the University of Minnesota found that soldiers refused to choke down more than one repast based on the unappealing blend. Keys then quickly proposed his own version of the "shirt-pocket meal," culling the ingredients from the shelves of a nearby grocery store: dry sausage (later a small can of processed meat), soy-flour biscuits (these gave a major leg up to the soybean industry after the war), a chocolate bar, and hard candy (later jazzed up with cigarettes, chewing gum, and toilet paper). Everything except for the meat was wrapped in cellophane, a transparent, cellulose-based packaging film invented in Switzerland at the turn of the century, and then packed into a flat cardboard box; the whole thing weighed only twelve ounces. This became the K ration, notable for being the first army food not universally reviled by soldiers.

Thus, when the United States officially entered the war on December 8, 1941, the day after Pearl Harbor was bombed by the Japanese, the Quartermaster Corps was ready. Sort of.

Troops, their numbers climbing to almost four million, were dispersed to practically every corner of the globe: the Pacific islands, North Africa, Europe, the Middle East, Australia, and even the Alaska Territory. This put American-made military supplies to the test, which they didn't always pass: tents rotted, boots felt apart, and canned rations rusted. Moreover, poor food allegedly had a role in one of the war's most devastating defeats. In the Philippines, seventy-six thousand U.S. and Filipino troops, low on rations and ammunition, surrendered to the Japanese in April 1942 and were forced to march across the Bataan Peninsula to prisoner camps. At least fifty-two hundred Americans died during the journey. One soldier who survived, an MIT graduate named Samuel Goldblith, helped to keep himself and fellow inmates healthy by drinking juice squeezed from grass and devised a vitamin A deficiency test by measuring a subject's ability to see light through sheets of toilet paper. He later became a professor in MIT's Department of Food Technology.

In the hand-wringing and finger-pointing that followed, the Quartermaster Corps' entire research program (or lack thereof) came under fire. Until then, new items had been developed sporadically and without coordination at four separate depots—shoes in Boston, clothing in Philadelphia, tents in Jefferson, Indiana, and food in Chicago. Responsibility for research was abruptly wrenched from the drowsy depots and centralized in Washington, D.C., at the Research and Development Branch of the Quartermaster's Military Planning Division, a new agency created in July 1942 to streamline planning, production, and distribution.

★ ★ ★

IN 1940 GEORGES DORIOT, a Harvard Business School professor of French origin, was looking for a way to contribute to the war effort. So when

Quartermaster General Edmund Gregory, who'd attended one of his classes a few years earlier, invited him to join the corps, he jumped at the chance, relocating to the nation's capital for the duration. In 1941 he was assigned to his first post, overseeing vehicle manufacturing, a familiar enterprise because Doriot had been groomed to take over his father's car-manufacturing company, a plan derailed by his studies at Harvard and subsequent recruitment to teach a manufacturing course there. He was quickly promoted, and when the Quartermaster Corps revamped in the wake of Pearl Harbor, it was clear that he was the man to run the new Research and Development Branch.

In addition to instituting his management philosophy of leading through inspiration rather than exhortation and surrounding himself with a cadre of "high-ranking civilians"[5] to bypass typical hierarchical military decision making, Doriot took a new tack in product development, placing the soldier front and center. He talked to those who'd experienced extreme conditions—say, for example, to Arctic explorers about sleeping bags. He then consulted with scientists and engineers to best understand technical requirements and limitations. And after a prototype had been made, he gathered evaluations from users and first-hand observers. During Doriot's first year on the job, he replaced tin with plastic in clothing, shoes, and gear; set up a climatology lab; and sent gear testers for a ten-week camping trip to Mount McKinley in Alaska. Then, in December 1942, he was given the responsibility for developing food, a move that effectively demoted Isker. Doriot's new Subsistence Section in the Washington office and its oversight committee, the Subsistence Research Projects Board, would from now on direct research activities in the Chicago lab.

For the army, it was none too soon. By 1943 the number of enlisted men and women reached almost nine million, still island-hopping in the Pacific and finally starting to push back the Axis in Europe. For the Quartermaster Corps, it was a time of firsts: the first time warfare had been so mobile, the first time a war was fought in multiple climates, and "the first time in history large groups of men lived for long periods of time solely on commercially produced and processed foods."[6] These were not faring well. Reports were filtering back of soldiers who would rather go hungry than eat rations and of uneaten rations piled in trash heaps and littering roadways. "It is our opinion that the most critical and urgent problems are in the food field," said Doriot, in a 1944 speech to the National Academy of Sciences, "and it is there that the bulk of our attention will be focused."[7] In time-honored pass-the-buck fashion, he then blamed the food industry: "It is because so little has been done in a scientific way on foods before the war [by his calculations, the industry spent just 2 percent of revenues on research], that we now find that so many unsolved problems confront us."[8] Applying the methods of good manufacturing—the very things he'd taught to future captains of industry at Harvard Business School—to army food became his mantra, one fully supported by the Subsistence Board, which included the chastened Isker as well as Bernard Proctor of MIT, Ancel Keys, and many others from academia, government, and industry. "In carrying out its mission the laboratory would act 'as the hitherto missing military link between research groups and production groups,'"[9] averred Proctor, the man who would become its supervisor.

★ ★ ★

BERNARD PROCTOR WAS A CLASSIC MIT GEEK. Born in nearby Malden, he headed to Cambridge to rack up an S.B. (1923), a Ph.D. (1927), an assistant professorship (1930), and an associate professorship (1937), all in food technology, which was at the time a subdiscipline of the Biology and Public Health Department. In 1913 MIT had been one of the first two universities nationwide to offer courses in food science; the other was Oregon State University. (More than two decades later, that number had increased only slightly to five.) In 1937 Proctor published the first book on the subject, the rather unimaginatively titled *Food Technology*, with Samuel Prescott, whose seminal work on thermal death times, which established the time and temperature needed to kill different kinds of food-borne bacteria, had finally relieved consumers of the nagging fear of loss of life and limb from exploding tins of lobster and tomatoes. That same year, he and Prescott also organized the first meeting of what would become food science's most important trade association, attracting more than five hundred people. At the second conference two years later, attended by an even larger crowd, the Institute of Food Technologists (IFT) was formally established and its first leaders elected— Prescott as president and a Swift research scientist, Roy Newton, as vice president. Nonetheless, MIT's food technology division, housed in the nation's foremost factory of serious science guys and eager-beaver engineers, suffered from an inferiority complex.

Then came the war. In addition to his appointment to the Quartermaster committee, Proctor was enlisted to travel the country in 1943 as an expert consultant on food to Henry Stimson, the secretary of war. A year later, he was made full professor at MIT and was offered a job as director of subsistence and packaging research in Washington, with responsibility for "all food supply and ration development for the Army."[10] This meant supervising the Subsistence Research Laboratory—for which "creating [product] specifications was one of the most important and time-consuming tasks"[11]—running field and nutritional tests; overseeing research projects at universities and federal agencies and in industry; and coordinating with the food agencies of the Allies. While there, however, he didn't neglect his buddies back home. From July 1942 until after the end of the war, the Division of Food Technology did nothing but work on Quartermaster Corps contracts, including ones for dehydrated mashed potato powder; high-calorie, long-shelf-life emergency biscuits; precooked, frozen foods; a liquid ration for life rafts; and synthetic vitamin A.

The C; the D, a deliberately unpalatable chocolate bar for emergencies; and the K rations (both the A, fresh foods, and the B, prepared foods for consumption in camp, were not field rations) were microbiologically safe, but they looked and tasted awful. The canned meat and vegetables turned gray. The fat separated and went rancid. The meat tasted as if it had been cooked for months. Eggs and dairy were downright stinky. The cans themselves were weighty and unwieldy; light and flexible cellophane could only be used for dry foods. And provisions that might have been gobbled down without a second thought under normal circumstances became unappealing or even repugnant to soldiers who were agitated, exhausted, afraid, or fighting in extremely hot, cold, or humid conditions. The solution? Another committee.

In response to a request by Doriot, a special advisory group, the Committee on Quartermaster Problems, was formed in 1943 by the National Academy of Sciences–National Research Council (NAS-NRC) to address the myriad inadequacies of soldier supplies. (After the war, it became the Advisory Board on Quartermaster Research and Development; later still, as the Advisory Board on Military Personnel Supplies, it oversaw the Natick Center until 1984.) The group had four standing subcommittees for textiles, plastics, leather and footwear, and germicides, and dealt with subsistence projects on a case-by-case basis. (A Subcommittee on Food was added after the war.) As an entity of the National Academy of Sciences, it was supposed to promote good science and high professional standards, a goal shared by Bernard Proctor. The Subsistence Laboratory's external research program began to reflect this new orientation, favoring academic and institutional research over that of industry.

By 1944, as the tides of war were turning, the U.S. Armed Forces surged to 11.4 million, and on June 6 the Allies invaded German-held France. Although they suffered heavy casualties, they were able to retake Paris. From a larger space, the newly designated Quartermaster Subsistence Research and Development Laboratory had added several menu items and two rations for small groups of soldiers, the 10-in-1 and the 5-in-1—extralarge cans of meat combinations packed with sides, utensils, and condiments—to its wares, which met with a better reception from the troops. Under Proctor's sure hand, with the help of a new addition to the Washington office, Emil Mrak, and the tireless ministrations of Isker, the lab had grown from the small, ill-equipped office it had been at the start of the war to become the administrative hub for food research undertaken all over the country, as well as a busy center in its own right where chemical, bacteriological, vitamin, and other studies were carried out. A food acceptance laboratory was added, headed by the University of Maine biologist W. Franklin Dove, to work full-time on understanding soldiers' eating preferences; tracking consumer food habits, one of its practices, has since become an industry standard. "We worked out methods to test for acceptability, involving color, flavor, texture, noise—potato chips have to make a noise, you don't like a potato chip that doesn't make a noise—pain—chili con carne—tackiness in peanut butter," said Mrak. "There were some seventeen factors that would come in, including heat, cold and rancidity, into food acceptance."[12]

The climax came the next year. In April 1945 the Soviet Union advanced into Berlin, and Hitler did what all (dis)honorable dictators do when cornered: he fled—in his case, this mortal coil, by committing suicide in an underground bunker and then having his followers burn the remains. Although the battle still waged in the Pacific, the European war was all but over. The number of troops was at its apogee, 11.6 million, as was the size of the Subsistence Research and Development Laboratory. By July 1945 it had 284 staff, hundreds of food and packaging projects, and innumerable cooperative relationships—both formal and informal—with universities, companies, and other government agencies. Proctor, while continuing to serve as consultant to the army, returned to Boston and civilian life, bringing with him a juicy irradiated food sterilization project that would be his program's primary source of income for more than two decades. Unperturbed, the army tapped one of MIT's rising rivals, the University of California, to carry on its food research program.

★ ★ ★

EMIL MRAK CAME FROM HUMBLE BEGINNINGS. A farmer's son, he entered the field of food technology—according to him, the discipline was started to employ jobless enologists during Prohibition—because he didn't see a future in agriculture. At the University of California, he fell hard—for yeasts, on which he wrote his thesis. After graduation, however, he returned to his fruit-growing roots, becoming a prune fellow, a position funded by the California Prune and Apricot Growers Association. While there, he answered such pressing questions as whether or not prunes had a "laxative principle" (they do) and if they were detectable in the urine of San Quentin inmates (they are; why the association cared remains unanswered). Another of Mrak's early academic achievements was the substitution of V8 juice for the gypsum blocks used for sporulating yeasts. But his carefree days among the microbes were numbered.

Mrak's first Quartermaster Corps project was studying how to dehydrate fruits and vegetables without deterioration from yeast, mold, or browning, an assignment given to the university because his mentor and thesis adviser, William Cruess, was a pioneer in the field. He also participated in the Quartermaster committees and was eventually invited by Proctor's colleague W. Ray Junk to "come on back and work with us."[13] After Proctor's departure at the tail end of 1944, Mrak moved to Washington. "I was asked to assume chairmanship of a newly created committee, entitled the Committee on Food Research, which was to develop external research programs relating to various foods used in rations, to hold symposia, to call on scientific personnel throughout the country for help, and so on. . . . [The office was] probably 250 feet long, and fifty or sixty feet wide, with tiny little desks about half the size of an ordinary desk so you always had to have stuff on the floor. . . . It was a temporary— what I call a permanent temporary building. . . . There must have been twenty or thirty people in this office, and at one end was a little office— a very small one where Ray Junk was (then it was Captain Junk)—and beyond him was Dr. Bernie Proctor's office. Upstairs was the same setup, but up there was Colonel McClain. . . . Colonel McClain was the guardian, or the gatekeeper for the General [Doriot]. So, if you wanted anything out of the General, you had to go through the Colonel."[14] By midyear 125 projects in eighty-four laboratories had been begun; seven conferences on topics such as the deterioration of fats and oils, food habits, developing concepts of protein metabolism, metabolism of low-caloric intake, bread staling, microbiology, and dairy chemistry had been organized; and numerous publications had been issued.

By July 1945 the Americans had retaken the Philippines, but heavy casualties were predicted for the final assault on Japan. Weary of the bloodshed, the United States decided to detonate the deadly flowers of its war science program. World War II ended with two giant booms: the vaporizing blasts in Hiroshima on August 6 and Nagasaki on August 9.

Victory was ours, but it had been a herculean effort. It wasn't that the United States had been unprepared for a global war. After being caught almost empty-handed when World War I erupted, the army had spent two decades coming up with the rapid, large-scale mobilization plan that had guided the country's efforts as it scaled up to join the multinational scrum. But even this preparation hadn't been enough to forestall or curtail the unprecedented cost and loss of human life.

The lesson of World War II was clear: We needed more. Bigger budgets. Longer time lines. Better training. Closer cooperation. In a word—one originally proposed by President Theodore Roosevelt—more *preparedness.* (The concept also does a great job at keeping the military employed during interwar periods—the five American wars since 1945 only kept the Defense Department busy about half the time.) The immediate postwar period may have seen a military demobilization, but in the sciences, the government was already building up for the next big engagement—by order of Army Chief of Staff Dwight D. Eisenhower. "The Army as one of the main agencies responsible for the defense of the nation has the duty to take the initiative in promoting closer relations between civilian and military interests. It must establish definite policies and administrative leadership which will make possible even greater contributions from science, technology, and management than during the last war."[15]

This postwar science policy fit perfectly with the army's already greatly increased investment in basic and applied food research—all it had to do was make the program begun in early 1945 and spearheaded by Mrak known to the public. Army public relations experts placed articles in papers around the country explaining the program's mission to find solutions for things like gray hash and stale bread. "The war produced atomic fission and radar, but no substitute for hardtack, it turns out."[16] An investment in food research was especially politically appealing in the wake of wartime and postwar food shortages in the United

States and abroad. Forty-four years later, Samuel Goldblith, the Bataan Death March hero who became an MIT food technology professor, commented, "This external research program was really the beginning of the major external R&D support at universities throughout the country, with federal government funding. A number of leading lights (and others who would become leading lights) in food technology were on temporary duty spearheading the Quartermaster Corps research and development effort. These men, who were then in their forties, included such luminaries as Bernard Proctor, Emil Mrak, W. Ray Junk, Samuel Lepkovsky, Rohland Isker, and M.L. (Tim) Anson, to name but a few. The Quartermaster Corps' R&D effort was important per se, but it also assumed long-range importance by being an important catalyst to the emergence of food science as a discipline in the United States."[17]

★ ★ ★

NINE MONTHS AFTER PEACE WAS DECLARED, Rohland Isker retired from the army, and the Subsistence Research and Development Laboratory, newly christened the Food and Container Institute for the Armed Forces, entered its final professional-scientist phase. It may have been that Isker was ready for a change—after all, he'd already served the requisite thirty years to receive a full pension. Or it may have been suggested that there was no longer a need for the sort of impromptu management style he'd perfected during the crisis in comestibles. But the directorship was obviously a role that Isker was reluctant to relinquish, and he quickly turned to his one remaining resource—an address book bulging with important industrial names—to re-create something of the power and excitement of the war years. In 1946, he founded a trade association, the Associates of the Food and Container Institute for the Armed Forces, which, within a year, had 166 food and packaging industry members. The group's executive officers were from American Can Company, General Foods, Armour, Swift, and others of that ilk and declared their intention to "serve as a clearing house for policy decisions concerning research required for the food and container industry of the Armed Forces."[18] In August 1948 Clarence Francis, chairman of General Foods, who had been Roosevelt's war production facilities manager, was appointed its chairman. While this organization never achieved the scientific spark-plug role Isker envisioned for it, it's lasted for sixty years, principally as a way for smaller contractors to win army ration procurement contracts.

When the war ended, Georges Doriot also put to good use his new knowledge and extensive connections, becoming the "Father of Venture Capitalism." He founded the American Research and Development Corporation (ARDC) to "furnish capital to companies principally engaged in the development of new enterprises, processes and new products"[19] and, with an exemption from the Securities and Exchange Commission (SEC), began offering stock in it to the public right away. ARDC, presided over by Doriot, also had on its board of directors MIT's president, Karl Compton, as well as several other professors from the institute. How important were Doriot's years in Washington with the Quartermaster Corps to this enterprise? His biographer, Spencer Ante, says, "It was through World War II that he underwent the most significant metamorphosis of his life, transforming himself from a professor of business into a world-class builder of innovative new enterprises. When Doriot became head of the Military Planning Division in the Office of the Quartermaster General, he began running, in a sense, his first venture capital operation."[20]

Bernard Proctor and Emil Mrak returned to their respective campuses to found two of the nation's most important food technology programs—at least until MIT pulled the plug on theirs in the 1980s, due to dwindling federal grant monies for the field. Both men continued to be active in military-funded research—Proctor worked primarily on irradiation of food and Mrak on yeasts—and both rose to become administrators in their universities. Each man served as president of IFT, the organization that Proctor and his mentor Samuel Prescott had helped to form right before the war. Today the organization has more than twenty-one thousand members worldwide; it serves both as a nexus for the industry through its meetings and widely attended annual conference and as an important source of information on food research through its various publications. In addition, after the war, Mrak's colleague from the

Committee on Food Research and editor of *Advances in Protein Chemistry,* Harvard professor Mortimer Anson, recommended him to his publisher, Academic Press. With this support, Mrak founded the influential *Advances in Food Research;* many of the studies highlighted in its early issues had been done or funded by the armed forces or other government agencies working in collaboration with them. Marveled Mrak thirty years later: "That Committee on Food Research, the Quartermaster laboratory in Chicago, and now that laboratory at Natick, Massachusetts (one I'm still advisor to), have benefitted the civilian population more than will ever be known. A lot of the foods we have today, the idea of acceptability and convenience, and stability, all came out of the war, the Quartermaster Corps. They're still producing new things that people use; the average citizen doesn't know this."[21]

★ ★ ★

IN THE UNIVERSE OF PROCESSED FOOD, World War II was the Big Bang. A blazing maelstrom of particles and energy, impenetrable to the observer, that as they cooled and drifted apart formed stars, planets, moons, and wandering clouds of dust. The sun is the Natick Center (first the Subsistence Research Laboratory and then the Quartermaster Food and Container Institute for the Armed Forces), the source of many, if not most, of the new scientific concepts and major technological breakthroughs that go into making everything from morning coffee to late-night chocolate chip cookies. The planets and moons are the Institute of Food Technologists, the world's biggest food technology trade association, a streamlined way to disseminate and exchange information, and a broad network of university food technology departments, most of which have been employed directly by DOD on one project or another and all of which teach new generations of students the knowledge mined for decades by the Natick Center. And the clouds of wandering dust? The myriad companies whose products—built on that same knowledge—are the ones we reach for day in and day out in our kitchens, at the minimart, and in the grocery store.

Chapter 7

WHAT AMERICA RUNS ON

LUNCH BOX ITEM #1: ENERGY BARS

It's Saturday morning, and cleats clatter up and down the stairs.

I'm still in bed sipping the cup of motor oil–strength coffee my husband has placed on the bedside table.

"Did you comb your hair?" I shout through the closed door. "Brush your teeth? Put on sunscreen? Do you have your water bottle? What'd you eat for breakfast?"

"A granola bar," yells Dalila from the bathroom where, octopus-like, she's complying with my grooming requests. A car pulls up outside. More clattering.

"Have a great game!" She's off.

Is there any quicker fix than an energy bar? These bars are the leitmotif of my daughters' childhoods. I'm always removing half-eaten bars from backpacks, coat pockets, lunch boxes, and purses, amazed that no matter how long they've been there, they're never stale or moldy. I find the shiny, foil-lined polypropylene wrappers—which I try to avoid reading; how many sugar variations can you fit in one product?—under beds, in corners, beside the sofas, and, occasionally, in the trash. The treats go with us everywhere: soccer practice, gymnastics class, dance class, nature hikes, the beach, and long car rides. In memory, their faintly sweet smell is almost indistinguishable from that of my children's breaths—pre–dental decay, pre–bad habits—as they dozed off in their car seats or strollers, the snack clutched in their chubby fists. The bars seemed as innocent as they were.

TOSSED INTO GLOVE COMPARTMENTS and office desk drawers. Tucked into backpacks and gym totes. Stowed in handbags and briefcases. Buried in kitchen cabinets. And, of course, sold by the boxful at every mini-mart, gas station, and supermarket from Bangor to Juneau, San Diego to Orlando. It's probably no exaggeration to say that the average American is never farther than twenty feet away from an energy bar (or, as they are variously called, granola bar, cereal bar, breakfast bar, nutrition bar, health bar, protein bar, sports bar, or snack bar). The small, flat rectangles of grains and vegetable or dairy protein, bound together with copious sugary syrup, are a fixture of modern-day eating: quick, portable, and (supposedly) nutritious, generating $5.7 billion in sales in 2011. We consume them as meals, in-between meals, and sometimes as dessert. But for all its ubiquity, the energy bar is a newcomer to our diet, making its first appearance in the 1970s and still a novelty by the mid-1990s, the freakish fare of will-deficient dieters and dangerously ardent athletes. From where did it come and why did it take us by storm?

The energy bar story begins a century ago, when the U.S. Army sought to turn chocolate, the world's favorite sweet, into an emergency ration for tired soldiers on the move. Being the army, however, it wasn't content just to serve what was already the perfect pick-me-up. It had to meddle and, in signature fashion, took on the two qualities that make chocolate chocolate: its delicious taste and its almost-body-temperature melting point. The fatty fruit of the *Theobroma cacao* tree, when ground, dissolves at between 93°F and 98°F, which means it tarries on the tongue, spreading and aerating over six hundred flavor compounds in a heady ooze. For three centuries after chocolate's discovery in the New World, only the rich could afford the fermented, roasted, and milled beans, which they used to make a hot beverage by mixing with water or milk and another irresistible—but expensive—tropical transplant, sugar. By the mid-1800s, sugar production had spread far and wide, and its price had dropped, leaving in its wake terrible teeth, spreading middles and backsides, and the forced resettlement of millions of Africans to charming beachfront properties throughout the Caribbean and the Americas. But no matter how cheap its principal ingredient, there's only so much hot cocoa a person can drink.

It took the Industrial Revolution, when machines were introduced for pressing powder from the nibs, to unlock the secret to producing solid chocolate. The process left behind prodigious quantities of an oily goop called cocoa butter, and manufacturers, always keen to find a market for industrial waste, hit upon the idea of mixing it back into the sugar-sweetened powder. This made a viscous liquid that could be formed into different shapes as it cooled. Candy! (The conche, another invention of the industrial age, crushed and agitated the blend, giving modern-day chocolate its delectable smoothness.) At first, hardened chocolate was used most often as a coating to create bonbons, which were downed, daintily but unceasingly, by the fairer sex festering in her domestic prison. But the treats, which were bought at the confectioner's, were still expensive and, what with their association with ladies who lunch, considered sissy food by half the adult population.

Until Milton S. Hershey came along.

By the age of thirty, Hershey had founded a successful caramel company (the main ingredients were imported sugar and milk from the state's one million hyperlactating—descriptor of the Department of Agriculture—cows) in Lancaster, Pennsylvania, but he was hungry for more. At the 1893 Chicago World's Fair, he saw some German chocolate-making machinery and decided to give the newfangled process a whirl. Six years later, he sold off the caramel branch of his business and committed himself full-time to producing cocoa, bonbons, syrup, and—finally—bars made from a secret Swiss procedure he'd painstakingly replicated. By substituting a cheap local ingredient—milk—for part of the expensive, imported one—cacao—he was able to make a chocolate candy that was affordable for all (and, with its masculine rectangle, far less threatening to the male ego than the bosomy bonbons of yore). Of course, this technique essentially turned the namesake ingredient into a flavoring agent, because it now made up, and still does, only 11 percent of the whole, but who's complaining when you're talking about five-cent candy bars? (The nickel bar didn't vary in price for almost seven decades; it just got smaller and smaller, until it vanished in a puff of smoke on November 4, 1969, the point at which it became impossible to turn a profit from it.) By the end of the first decade of the twentieth century, the Hershey bar was sold in every corner store, newsstand, and lunch counter across the country, and its inventor was so rich he built two company towns, one in Pennsylvania and the other in Cuba.

The U.S. military had taken notice not only of the world's growing infatuation with the Mesoamerican food of the gods but also of the fact that German researchers heralded the sugar-laden bars as a better alternative to alcohol—prohibited in the American military since 1832—in stimulating men for long hikes and grueling manual labor. By the late 1890s the army was experimenting with a new emergency ration that included the mood-elevating sweet as well as a knockoff of the indigenous North American road fuel, pemmican, a mouthwatering mixture of pulverized meat and maize in animal fat. It contracted with two companies, the ephemeral American Compressed Food Company and Armour & Company (the latter brand still does business with Uncle Sam as Pinnacle Foods and Smithfield Foods and has had its greedy fingers in every war pie made since its founding in 1867). The army performed what passed for taste testing at the time: sending a bunch of guys to the woods with the new rations to see what stuck. Both prototypes were found lacking. According to the report, "Everybody suffered excessively from hunger, and in spite of the surreptitious begging of food from camping parties, the greater part of the men were reduced to a pitiable state of weakness."[1]

Not to be deterred, the army vowed it would devise its own emergency ration, which it did, debuting in 1910 an all-in-one chocolate number that included egg albumin and nucleo-casein for protein and stability. Reactions were still less than enthusiastic—the item apparently provoked nausea and dizziness, and the secretary of war halted the project in 1913. Although the Department of Agriculture's Bureau of Nutrition Investigations then came up with a slightly more palatable version, when preparations for World War I began, the army still hadn't found a lightweight, energy-packed battle ration that could be carried in a pocket and eaten on the move.

The war to end all wars broke out, as so many conflicts have, in the Balkans, from where it spread quickly to infect all of Europe with a nasty case of trench warfare. Deep in their warren of dugouts, tunnels, and channels, when soldiers weren't busy snoozing in the mud, waving off rats, and tossing grenades, they worked their way through piles of rations. First off, the Trench, with canned meat or fish and hard bread, as well as cigarettes and solidified alcohol for up to twenty-five troops. After that, the Reserve, which provided a day's worth of canned meat, hard bread, sugar, and coffee for one man. When things got really desperate, they dreamed of chocolate . . . and had another Reserve. Having resoundingly rejected Armour's can full of pemmican-lite and chocolate candy (three packets of each) almost two decades earlier, the Quartermaster Corps hadn't placed its wartime order until June 6, 1918. It arrived too late. Five months later, on November 11, 1918, the day the Allies and Germany signed the armistice, the first one million emergency rations, with their payloads of half sugar, half chocolate made by the venerable New York chocolatier Maillard Chocolate Manufacturers, were still floating across the Atlantic Ocean. (The surplus was later sold at below cost to Boy Scouts, hunters, explorers, and others.)

Of course, gastronomic suffering wasn't limited to the Western Front. At home, Americans were asked to make sacrifices, too, going meatless on Monday and wheatless on Wednesday, and limited to just eight ounces of sugar per week. Industry's use of the sweetener was also rationed; only commercial fruit preservers, vegetable packers, milk condensers, jam manufacturers, ice-cream makers, and military contractors could buy as much as they wished. Confectioners, on the other hand— yet to convince the public that snacks were a valid fifth food group—were cut to just 50 percent of their previous year's purchase and scolded for their hoarding ways. In a 1919 memo, George Zabriskie, president of the U.S. Sugar Equalization Board, which controlled distribution and set prices for the commodity, noted acidly: "Our observation has been that candy manufacturers have not only had their normal supply of sugar, but in many cases have anticipated their wants and been able to acquire sugar ahead of more essential industries."

Much to his dismay, that didn't include Milton Hershey, who by then owned an entire Monopoly board of assets, including numerous properties in the United States and Cuba, multiple residences for himself and executives, worker housing, mills, factories, schools, stores, parks, and even railroads. Hershey—horrors!—was unable to obtain sufficient sugar to keep vendors stocked with candy. This was not at all satisfactory, especially because competitors on the military payroll faced no such restrictions. (It was at this point that strapped chocolate makers began mixing in breakfast cereals, dried fruit and cookies, giving rise to such delicacies as Mars Mounds and the Nestlé Crunch bar.) Hershey vowed he would not again get stuck on the outside looking in during wartime.

His chance came when the army decided to have another go at the emergency ration—but instead of providing three separate components, it would combine protein, carbohydrate, and sweet in one. Mind you, this couldn't be too tasty, or the men wouldn't bother waiting for a crisis to eat them. In 1937, after two years of internal research, Colonel Paul Logan of the U.S. Army Quartermaster Corps, the head of the Subsistence School, began looking for a company foolhardy enough to take on stripping the pleasure from one of humankind's most seductive foods by reengineering it so that the candy wouldn't melt in pockets or at tropical temperatures or be overly tempting to sweet-toothed soldiers. He didn't need to look far; Hershey, now the nation's largest chocolate factory, jumped at the opportunity—being part of the rations supply chain would mean its sugar-gluttonous manufacturing line would never be subject to wartime restrictions again.

Logan provided his patented formula—about one-third bitter chocolate, one-third sugar, one-sixth skim milk powder, one-fifteenth oat flour, and a few vanillin crystals—for making a barely edible chocolate bar, and after a few days of trial runs in the Hershey lab, it was approved for production. The dough was so thick it had to be pressed into the molds by hand. The finished bars were sealed in foil and then paper-wrapped in sets of three, for a total of 1,800 calories, enough to sustain a man for one day. (Later, when foil became scarce during World War II and the use of chemical weapons seemed imminent—mustard and chlorine gas had been used frequently in World War I—waterproof cellophane and wax-coated boxes were used.) The so-called Logan bar, or D ration, was, by all accounts, awful. Nonetheless, between 1941 and 1944, almost a quarter billion bars were shipped and stockpiled overseas,[2] and Hershey was basking in its new role as premier chocolatier to the U.S. Army.

This Frankenchoc—part protein, part grain, and a helluva lot of $C_{12}H_{22}O_{11}$—was the great-granddaddy of the modern energy bar, and has gone to war in soldiers' pockets in every American military engagement up until the Gulf War. After World War II, there was a gradual split in the evolutionary tree, with the energy bar becoming a cereal-based meal-in-a-fist while nonmelting chocolate returned to its candy roots. But although billions have been produced, the waxy, cacao-based confection never gained any admirers. Hershey tweaked the D ration formula a couple of times. It began making the ever-so-slightly tastier Tropical Bar in 1943 for use in the hot and humid Pacific theater. This recipe was dusted off during the Korean War (1950–53) and the early years of Vietnam involvement (starting in 1955). Oat flour was eliminated in 1957, and the skim-milk powder replaced with nonfat milk solids (the difference between them is in the proportions of protein, lactose, and minerals). For the next several decades, Hershey complacently churned out this slightly, but obviously not much, improved candy. According to a Vietnam-era report, "Mother Bollman hands out bars of Hershey's Tropical Chocolate for breakfast on the morning of the last day of the patrol. . . . For us, [they] are a last resort. They'll provide some energy and a little bit of a needed sugar boost, but they'll also require a swallow or two of our remaining water to wash away the taste."[3]

But trouble was on the horizon. After decades of doldrums, progress was finally being made on producing a heat-tolerant chocolate. First Food-Tek, Inc., in New Jersey used polyhydric alcohols, an emulsifier that helped distribute the fat, and then the Battelle Memorial Institute, a longtime military contractor, in its Geneva laboratories, added water and a top-secret surfactant to increase the substance's melting point without—according to them—changing its quality. In the late 1980s, researchers at the Natick Center came up with a new formulation based on this concept—tentatively dubbed the Congo Bar—that could withstand up to 140°F, and asked Hershey to produce 144,000 bars for the 1990–91 Gulf War, and a second shipment of 750,000 units several months later. Press releases taunted rival Mars (makers of M&M's) that the Desert Bar was "a candy bar that melts in your mouth, not in the sand."[4] Mars, which had its eye on expanding its market in the Middle East, responded by going after Hershey's military business. When DOD put the next contract for the Desert Bar out to bid—some 6.9 million units—Mars won it. And like a decades-old marriage held together by inertia, the historic U.S. Army–Hershey relationship crumbled in an instant. (A resulting legal battle between the two chocolate giants was also won by Mars.) However, neither version of the Desert Bar was well liked, and neither made it to the commercial market.

The quest for heat-tolerant chocolate continues. In the early 2000s, Cadbury—owned by Mondelēz, the new Latinized Kraft moniker—found that reconching further broke down the sugar molecules, increasing the overall melting point of the sucrose-in-lipid suspension. And several manufacturers, including Barry Callebaut, experimented with fats—either drastically reducing the cocoa butter or adding in fats that are solid at room temperature. It may not be today, or even tomorrow, but when the breakthrough finally comes it will deliver a prize far larger than thousands of fatigue pockets and camouflage rucksacks: the 3.8 billion chocolate-deprived souls who live in those areas of the world still shockingly deficient in cold chains, continuous refrigeration systems—geographic footnotes such as Africa, Latin America, south and central Asia, and the Middle East.[5]

★ ★ ★

WHILE MELTLESS CHOCOLATE AMBLED OFF in a different direction, the idea of a fortified food bar, especially a sweetened one, lingered on, playing a starring role in two of the army's most important research programs of the 1950s, '60s, and '70s: freeze-drying and intermediate-moisture foods. When commercial versions finally began to emerge, they had tucked inside not only enough calories and nutrients to provide a jolt of cheap energy, but also several major breakthroughs in twentieth-century food science, courtesy of the Department of Defense.

Industrial freeze-drying wasn't born in the field kitchen but in the medic's tent. Historically, 90 percent of all war fatalities have taken place on the battlefield, most often from loss of blood. This all changed after World War I with the convergence of two discoveries. The first was the understanding that battlefield shock was not, as had been previously thought, a nervous system shutdown, but a circulatory slowdown caused by loss of blood volume. (Think of the difference in pressure between a trickle and a torrent of water from a garden hose.) This meant that doctors and nurses could skip whole-blood transfusions and just inject plasma, the clearish carrier fluid, to stave off the downward spiral to death. The second was a new contraption rigging together airtight chambers, vacuum pumps, and condensers that allowed large-scale freeze-drying in commercial labs. Now, not only could fallen men be treated for shock on the spot, but they could receive plasma that had been made into a powder, shipped thousands of miles, stored for months on end, and rehydrated as needed. A new age of battlefield medicine—indeed, of emergency medicine—was born. (It was brief. It turned out that freeze-drying also preserved plasma's scruffy viral hitchhikers, hepatitis B and, later, HIV; the use of pooled whole plasma was halted in 1968.)

Until the invention of freeze-drying, the only way to remove fluid from organic matter had been to allow its water to change from liquid to gas, either through a leisurely air-drying or a frenzied cooking. Both of these methods permanently alter tissues from prolonged exposure to oxygen or by denaturing proteins. But with lyophilization, for the first time, water could be dissipated while leaving cell walls and other structures uninjured. It works through a simple two-step process. The material is brought to below the freezing point, which slows down its molecules as if they had a major case of Parkinson's. Lacking the energy to escape, water molecules slip into fixed positions with their neighbors and ice crystals form in the material. Next, the pressure is drastically reduced. The vacuum forces the water molecules to suddenly relinquish their hold on their fellow H_2Os and others—sort of like abruptly encountering no resistance in an arm-wrestling match—and burst out of the surface of the ice. Whoosh! Vaporized. In no time at all, the vacuum arrives at the core of the frozen matter, stripping it of almost all its water. What's left behind is everything else, more or less intact. (Because water expands when it freezes, some slight damage is unavoidable.)

Freeze-drying's status as an unsung World War II hero—it indubitably rescued more fallen soldiers than all 464 of the Medal of Honor recipients combined—didn't stop the army from eyeballing the new preservation tool for more everyday ends: food. Foreseeing a tide that has yet to ebb, military analysts predicted a need for ever-greater troop mobility. And what would be more conducive to that than rations from which most of the weight, which is water, had been removed? Even at the beginning, however, there were signs that this decision was foolhardy. "The experience of World War II and Korea showed that dehydrated products were of questionable acceptability, and it was well known that the commercial sector had all but rejected dehydration as a viable process, [but] the Army still encouraged its proliferation," wrote Stephen Moody, director of the Natick Center's Combat Feeding Directorate, in his master's thesis.[6] Throughout the 1950s, the Quartermaster Food and Container Institute sponsored research on freeze-drying, mostly of meat, with contractors such as the University of California, Armour, the American Meat Institute Foundation, Rutgers, Oregon State, and the Georgia Institute of Technology, and also did its own in-house studies.

Liquids, such as coffee extracts, were relatively simple to preserve with the technique because they had no structural elements that needed to be maintained. Volatile compounds take longer to turn to vapor than water and some are trapped in the viscous coffee during the freeze-drying process. When the resulting powders, such as the instant Folgers and Sanka that so captivated our grandparents or the *café* in *café con leche*, are added to hot water, the aroma components are released again, giving the brew a reasonably good taste. But when things got more complicated than coffee or tea, the results were this side short of repulsive. Along with the water, the process ended up removing more of the volatiles, which escaped through cracks in the now brittle material, leaving food that tasted flat. Far worse was the impact on mouthfeel. Meat fibers were toughened; vegetable cellulose collapsed, ruptured by the ice crystals; and rehydration was fleeting—after the first bite, the fluid drained, leaving behind something resembling a damp loofah.

But the army wasn't discouraged; on the contrary, it was gung ho. In fact, by the late 1950s, armed forces subsistence experts had developed a delightfully futurist vision of on-the-go chow based on freeze-drying: there would be stacks of cute little bars, and soldiers would munch their way through three square meals plus snacks (or rehydrate them for a luxury dining experience)—breakfast cereal, bacon and eggs (scratch the eggs—stability problems), split pea soup, hash browns, fruit, carrots and peas, chicken and rice, fudge brownie. And to accommodate the human compulsion to customize, men could season to taste by tearing off a sheet from a booklet of laminated condiments: ketchup, barbecue sauce, sautéed onions, jams, peanut butter, soy sauce, maple syrup, and relish. But the military still didn't have the industrial base necessary to execute this sweeping plan. So the Quartermaster Food and Container Institute convened a conference in September 1960 on its efforts to create light, long-shelf-life rations. More than four hundred participants from government, industry, and academia attended, and less than a year later a second, more technically oriented international gathering was held to "lead to a more attractive economic outlook for freeze-dried foods."[7] Even so, this pie-in-the-sky project might have continued to languish, but for the fortuitous appearance of a real need for sci-fi-style feeding: the race to the moon.

The U.S. space program was born of the Cold War—a scientific bicep popping intended to intimidate the Soviets by putting a man in space. But by the time President Eisenhower founded the National Aeronautics and Space Administration (NASA) in 1958, the USSR had already beaten the United States to the cosmological punch. The year before, they'd plopped Sputnik, the first artificial satellite, into orbit, rattling DOD cages with (entirely prescient) fears of sky spying and cross-continental missile strikes. In 1961 our archenemy propelled a real live human being, twentysomething Yuri Gargarin, for a whirlwind, one-hour-and-forty-eight-minute spin around the world. Although the United States sent up its first astronaut for a fifteen-minute motor-revving display a month later, the score was an alarming two zip.

NASA's lengthy to-do list included figuring out what's for dinner when you're 238,900 miles from home. Not only did food have to be compact, lightweight—in the early days, every pound off the ground cost $100,000—and ready to eat, it had to be completely hygienic. (Food poisoning, with its attendant ejaculation of chunky fluids from digestive tract termini, was highly undesirable.) Thus, it makes sense that the organization chosen to develop nourishment for astronauts was the army, first through the Quartermaster Food and Container Institute in Chicago and later through its successor, the Natick Center. The challenges of preparing space food and rations were remarkably similar, although space travel had its unique menaces, such as clouds of astronaut-choking, console-clogging, zero-gravity crumbs. First out of the gate, the harebrained-sounding food-bar scheme, which NASA bought lock, stock, and barrel, although with a twist: bite-size cubes instead of bars to eliminate the potential hazard of deadly crumbs. The cubes debuted on a 1962 Project Mercury flight to less than enthusiastic reviews—"harsh" and "dry" were the exact words. The freeze-dried tidbits actually subtracted moisture during mastication, so they left space travelers with a major case of dry mouth.

Negative taste tests notwithstanding, Natick Labs was soon awash in astrodollars. Even in that most affectless of documents, the meeting minutes, it was hard to disguise their elation: "This overall area is being heavily funded. The sophisticated requirements of these food bars have never been considered before and necessitate considerable contractual and in-house work to advance the technology thereof." By 1963 not only were the army's own labs working around the clock (during most of the decade, it had ten full-time staff people dedicated to the project), but it was overseeing at least sixteen industry and academic contracts for related research, including ones with Pillsbury, Swift, Archer Daniels Midland (ADM), the University of Minnesota, and MIT. Most were for applied research, developing such things as binders to impart structure and strength, edible coatings to foil flaking and exclude moisture and oxygen, and moisture-mimicking additives to make the bars somewhat edible. This work resulted in many industry patents from the mid-1960s onward. The MIT contract, on the other hand, was for an important basic research question: why didn't freeze-dried foods taste good? The man Natick chose to unravel this knotty problem was an up-and-coming young professor named Marcus Karel.

MARCUS KAREL IS CUT from a fine twentieth-century cloth that has all but gone the way of the gramophone. Humble, hardworking, and deeply humanitarian, as a teenage member of a semiclandestine Zionist group he helped Jews escape his home country of Poland after World War II. He then emigrated himself, eventually getting a job as an assistant in the MIT packaging lab and entering its food technology doctoral program. By the late 1950s, he had graduated to studying the permeability of different kinds of plastic films to water and flavor and also discovered his life's work: understanding how water and oxygen affect chemical reactions in food. Karel successfully defended his thesis in 1960 and was offered a faculty position in the Department of Nutrition, Food Science, and Technology.

Vital to Karel's work—and food science in general—was the concept of water activity, a new way to understand how its molecules behave in a substance. Water is the major component of almost all food. We living things are full of it—animals, about 70 percent; plants, 80–90 percent— and so, naturally, are edibles. The high proportion of water facilitates a dizzying number of chemical reactions and biological processes. After death, this tissue continues to be highly chemically reactive, although functioning, absent cellular respiration, trickles to a halt (except for enzymatic reactions, which depend only on the presence of their substrates to work). The lack of defenses, both barrier and immunological, turns the nutrient-rich organic matter into a virtual bacteria and fungi magnet. But although moisture is definitely associated with spoilage, the amount of water in a food doesn't always predict whether it will go bad.

The conundrum was solved by William James Scott, an Australian bacteriologist at the Council for Scientific and Industrial Research, who, before World War II, had studied spoilage in chilled ox muscle for that country's beef exporters, and during the war worked to ensure the safety of the food Australia supplied to the Allies. Starting in 1953, he did a series of experiments, adding different amounts of solutes to a nutritious substrate and then, after a set time period, recording the number of organisms for two of mankind's bacterial baddies, *Staphylococcus aureus* and *Salmonella*. The solutes lowered the substrate's vapor pressure ratio, a standard chemistry measurement. (The vapor pressure of pure water shows how much force water molecules exert on the surrounding air at a given temperature. The vapor pressure of a food at that same temperature is lower, because some of the water molecules are bound to the food material. The vapor pressure ratio, called the water activity, or a_w, by food scientists, is the vapor pressure of the food material at a given temperature divided by the vapor pressure of pure water at that same temperature. The more strongly the water molecules are bound to the food material, the lower the water activity.) What Scott found was that there was a vapor pressure ratio below which the population growth of bacteria was virtually zero—0.85 for *S. aureus* and 0.90 for *Salmonella* and most others. (Yeasts and molds can survive down to 0.60.) In early 1957 Scott proposed a new theory, one in which microbial spoilage was related not to absolute water content but to the amount of water available—that is to say, not chemically bound to the food material—for microorganisms to perform vital life functions (ingestion, respiration, reproduction, excretion).

Karel became one of the earliest proponents of Scott's water activity theory. His Ph.D. student Ted Labuza recalls his final year as an undergraduate in MIT's Department of Nutrition, Food Science, and Technology: "I had taken a course . . . with him where he introduced the concept of water activity and the application of kinetics to food storage stability. At that time there were no textbooks with this concept. . . . He had just then gotten a grant from the U.S. Army Natick Labs and the air force to work on stability of military and space foods." Karel's first space program work enumerated the things that could go awry with deeply desiccated foodstuffs.[8] As it turns out, there were a lot.

First, enzymes, which are present in all animals, most plants, many microorganisms, and fresh products made of the same, weren't inactivated by freeze-drying. Unless they were denatured by heat or acidity, these specialized proteins kept on catalyzing chemical reactions, in some cases creating a dark pigment that resulted in unappetizing-looking edibles. On the other hand, discoloration due to the breakdown and recombination of sugars and amino acids, known as nonenzymatic, or Maillard, browning, was minimal in freeze-drying. The surprise was lipids, which, when left high and dry, reacted with oxygen, creating a rancid taste.

"The Karel lab was a primary group combining kinetics, water activity, and packaging engineering, and Marcus was the orchestra master," explains Labuza, who worked on several of Karel's projects on deteriorative reactions in dehydrated food, "and the players, his 'science children' went on in food engineering as faculty somewhere compounding the impact of what Karel taught them." In 1965 teacher and pupil attended the first-ever international conference on water activity in food, a life-changing event for Labuza. "The Natick Center was there; their representative was a guy named Harold Salwin. He'd done a study with cookies that stored them at different relative humidities and what he found was that at lower relative humidities, the shelf life was reduced because of the oxidation of lipids. I was quite interested in that and it became the basis of my Ph.D. thesis."

The two MIT academics also scored a major funding coup, snagging NASA contracts to continue Karel's work on flavor degradation in freeze-dried foods, as well as one "to design foods for the space program under contract to the U.S. Air Force, in a classified research program called Skylab. The idea was to come up with a bar of some sort and study the shelf life of it," explains Labuza. After that, there was no stopping them. In the course of a few years, in addition to other technical reports for Natick, the air force, and NASA, the pair published articles together on related topics in the *Journal of Food Science* (1966), *Cryobiology* (1967), *Journal of Agricultural and Food Chemistry* (1968), *Journal of the American Oil Chemists' Society* (1969, 1971), *Food Technology* (1970), and *Modern Packaging* (1971). In 1969 Labuza; Steven Tannenbaum, a colleague; and Karel made the crucial breakthrough that enabled food technologists to put Scott's 1957 theory to use: a mathematical model that mapped water activity, temperature, and different deteriorative reactions.[9] Water sorption isotherms, which are based on observational data of water activity for each food item under the varying conditions, finally allowed companies to accurately predict shelf life for their products. Says Labuza, "The importance of Natick was that they had the money. The work that they funded really set the basic principles."

★ ★ ★

COMPARED WITH THE LIMITED OPTIONS of the first space travelers, the Project Apollo (1968–72) astronauts enjoyed the equivalent of a groaning cruise ship buffet—everything from bacon and chicken sandwiches to potato salad and pineapple fruitcake. There was only one hitch: almost everything was still freeze-dried, either in rehydratable packets or ready-to-eat nuggets. Despite the vastly expanded offering, the reaction was about the same as it had been back in 1962: "Inflight nausea, anorexia and undesirable physiological responses experienced by some crewmen were believed to be partly attributable to the foods," said the NASA bio-medical report. (The rehydratable entrées were also tried out in Vietnam with even worse results—reconstituting your food with jungle water is never a good idea.) At this point, it would have been sensible for the army to be a mite worried. Almost two decades had passed, and they still hadn't been able to make freeze-dried rations that tasted good. But still the army persevered, albeit conceding that "the use of plasticizers seems essential to this development." Industry contracts were duly awarded.

But just in case, the Natick Center also hedged its bets with some-thing moist that didn't require as much expensive equipment as did freeze-drying: dog food. In the early 1960s, General Foods had applied Scott's water activity principle to a relatively low-risk market segment—canines—and launched a new shelf-stable patty of extruded animal and vegetable proteins. The army wasn't going to slip actual Gaines-burgers into the mess kit, but if they borrowed a technique here and there and applied it to people chow, who'd know? In 1965 the Committee on Ani-mal Products of the Advisory Board on Military Personnel Supplies had already directed that "more attention be given to investigations on pres-ervation of foods at 'intermediate' moisture levels." A first industry con-tract, with General Foods, had been completed by 1968, and Natick, the air force, and NASA were working hand in hand, "since such close coop-eration assists greatly in the coordination of the research." The next NASA contract looked at the deterioration of intermediate-moisture foods (IMFs) and named Ted Labuza, an up-and-coming young MIT professor, as principal investigator.

Until IMFs came along, preservation was a Goldilocks story without the "just right" option. There was canned, which was fairly tasty, but heavy. And there was dried, which was generally not so tasty, but light. IMFs usually have a lower water content than normal foods, so they weigh a little less; however, more important, they have significantly reduced water activity, generally between 0.6 and 0.9 (by contrast, the a_w of dried food is 0.2 or less), so bacteria simply can't reproduce in the numbers necessary for spoilage or illness. That means that although they are soft and humid, IMFs can be stored at room temperature for a long time with just regular packaging materials. This development made the military—and its friends in the food industry—very happy indeed.

The master-apprentice relationship has a predictable arc. Awestruck adulation. Amiable peers. And, finally, a battle in which the disciple proves himself worthy by besting his mentor. In 1971, when Labuza was denied tenure and departed for the University of Minnesota, he took some of MIT's prestigious NASA contracts—in which he'd undoubtedly preened and posed during hiring talks—with him. It wasn't a clean victory; Labuza had tried to get NASA to invest immediately in the new IMF technology, but he was told that the contracts to produce freeze-dried rations had already been signed for two years.[10] But the center of gravity for NASA-funded investigation of cutting-edge food-preservation techniques had shifted from the country's most glamorous technical institute to a staid but steady public research college—and that was probably the moment when the sun began to set for MIT's Department of Nutrition and Food Science.

That summer, Labuza had a major triumph: the Apollo 15 astronaut David Scott snacked in space on his intermediate-moisture apricot food bars, which had been manufactured by Pillsbury, by threading them through a circular port in his helmet.

Ground control: Are you eating a fruit bar?

Scott: I might have been eating a fruit bar. I really liked the fruit bars. Anytime that was break time was a good time to have the fruit bar and a drink of water.[11]

The University of Minnesota's press release emphasizes the snack's longevity. "This bar-like food, high in calories per unit of weight, lasts about 6 months without refrigeration." Reflects Labuza on his contribution to the breakthrough, "Marcus Karel and I were key in the understanding of water activity from a thermodynamic [perspective], not just bound vs. free water. . . . Our labs and Duckworth's [another food scientist] set the stage. . . . Most soft chewy bars are based on our work." Even the conservative Advisory Council to the Natick Combat Feeding Program could see the commercial potential. According to its 1972 minutes, "It is important to note that the characteristics of these food products also make them of great value to a wide variety of civilian food requirements."

Labuza's star was in full ascendance during the 1970s. Over the course of his almost ten-year contract between NASA and the University of Minnesota, he hammered the kinks out of IMFs, mostly by applying the same approaches taken by Karel a decade before with freeze-dried foods. Toward the end of the decade, Labuza tackled humectants, one of the most important ingredients for food preservation; these compounds, such as the polyhydric alcohols glycerol and sorbitol, both lower the water activity by binding water and also impart a sense of moistness and softness, making food more palatable. "Only sweet flavors ended up being made for the space flights," explains Labuza. "It's a lot more difficult to lower the water activity of foods without sugar. For example, the water activity in a piece of meat can be lowered by adding salts and sugars, but these change the flavor, often undesirably."

The food industry has frequently come under fire for its lavish use of these solutes, and, specifically, its extensive research on how to more skillfully manipulate the flavor enhancers to addict us to junk food. But there's another equally important, if not more important, reason to lace our breakfast cereal, bread, lunch meat, chips, soups, heat-and-serve meals, and cookies with salt and sugar. Our food is geriatric, and these two common chemicals do an ace job at mummifying and bestowing false youth—bright colors, firm shapes, soft textures—to edibles way past their prime.

The ability of sugar and salt to preserve food has been understood instinctually, if not scientifically, since people began to break out the Egyptian *bottarga* (dried and salted fish roe) and Roman honey-preserved dormice at parties. Over millennia, salt and sugar evolved from precious—

even miraculous—substances fit to pay soldiers, grace the tables of kings, or be meted out by apothecaries, to mundane items bought by the box and sack in any grocery store. The two compounds work similarly to reduce deteriorative chemical reactions and prevent microbial growth, although they have some striking differences. Salt is a mineral, an inorganic compound; electromagnetically charged; and impervious to temperature changes. Sugars (there are various kinds) are from plants, are organic compounds (with a carbon molecule skeleton), are not electromagnetically charged, and become more soluble (more can be dissolved in water) the warmer it is. But in food, they do more or less the same thing, which is to sop up water like molecular Bounty; this dramatically lowers the concentration of free H_2O molecules around any microbial spoilers or pathogens, which then have their insides sucked dry by the same cell-wall osmosis on which they depend for water and nutrients. Sugar and salt can also break the bonds holding together bacterial enzymes, which inactivates them, and even unravel their DNA.

But that's just the beginning. If there are two more successful multitaskers, they have yet to be discovered. Both make major contributions to texture. Salt extracts water, creating denser solids that have a satisfying snap. Ordinary sugar (sucrose, from sugarcane or sugar beets) plays both sides, endowing either plasticity or crunch (for example, soft cookie vs. hard), depending on its type, water activity, and processing technique, and increases the viscosity of liquids, giving body and mouthfeel to soft drinks and syrups. Sugar is a consummate makeup artist, touching baked goods with gold and adding shimmer to sauces and glazes. The duo also enable secondary flavors, from sugar's participation in the world-famous Maillard reaction to salt's willingness to act as a shill for the artificial flavors in and dusted on chips, nuts, pretzels, popcorn, and extruded snacks. And both are key to activating or controlling important processing techniques such as leavening, marinating, pickling, and freezing. Is it any wonder that when the food industry needs a preservative, humectant, volumizer, bulking agent, dispersant, or color stabilizer, it most often chooses these two natural chemicals that taste good, are dirt cheap, and have a history of safe use that dates back to before the birth of Jesus, Mohammed, or any other major-religion-founding prophet?

Back in Minnesota, Ted Labuza helped his industry colleagues develop and patent IMFs for the consumer market. "The military had hired Pillsbury to make the bars," he says. "Once they were made, the military released the information." Former *Journal of Food Science* editor Daryl Lund explains why: "Information was disseminated nearly immediately because Natick had an interest in IMFs for long-term storage, combat rations, etc. The fact is that they also wanted that information out because they wanted people to develop food that would have this kind of shelf life." Labuza gave generously of his time, consulting with Pillsbury (its 1970 Space Food Sticks may have been a little before the curve; they bombed), Quaker Oats, General Mills, and other companies. From the mid-1970s to early 1980s, a barrage of energy bars hit the market, all from large companies, many of them frequent Natick partners, including General Foods, Carnation, Kellogg's, Kraft, and Nabisco. Their target audience? "Mothers will be able to give their children sweet substitutes for candy that are highly balanced in protein, fat, sugar, and vitamins," explains Labuza.

Meanwhile, Marcus Karel, Labuza's former teacher, labored on in MIT's Nutrition and Food Science Department, which, observing waning Defense Department and NASA interest, had beefed up its nutritional research and thrown itself into global public health and the crowded National Institutes of Health ring, competing against a multitude of medical researchers. But despite its change in focus, the program began to fade; it lost the spotlight among the university's exemplary departments in annual reports, and the number of graduate students and undergraduate majors began to decline. Eventually MIT dismantled the whole operation, parceling out professors to other disciplines, retiring others, and, in an institutional sense, banishing food science to the kitchen to scour pots while inviting its former colleagues chemistry, biology, and engineering to feast in the dining room.

And what became of the army's double-decade-long, multimillion-dollar investment in freeze-drying? The military quietly changed course and hoped no one would remember the minilibrary of dehydrated, compressed bars it envisioned each soldier would have buried in her rucksack. In the commercial market, the forlorn remnants of this once-bright technology are found in your favorite déclassé breakfast: instant coffee and cold cereal studded with nibs of dried strawberries, raspberries, or blueberries.

★ ★ ★

IF YOU COULD TRAVEL BACK IN TIME TO 1983, it's doubtful you would have picked three underachieving or unemployed Frisco runners (a biophysics and medical physics Ph.D., a recently fired track and field coach, and a nutrition student) as the trio who would allay one of the nation's most deep-seated anxieties, that of engaging in everyday activities without a stockpile of snacks. That year, Brian Maxwell, who six years earlier had blazed to third place in the Boston Marathon, hit the wall in a small race. The wall is the point around the twenty-mile mark when the little orange light starts to glow on the gas gauge: the body has used up all its available blood glucose, stored glycogen, and fats (fats are even less available during intense physical activity because muscles must tie up much of their oxygen to metabolize them). Doubled over in pain, he completed the course, but lost his position as a front-runner. A die-hard competitor, Maxwell vowed never again. He set about creating a lightweight, nutritionally balanced snack that would restore lost vitamins, minerals, and amino acids and provide the perfect punch to finish the race.

Over the next few years, Maxwell, Bill Vaughan, and Jennifer Biddulph, Maxwell's future wife and a nutrition student, munched on enough not-quite-right energy bars to last several lifetimes. The process was fetchingly homespun: They concocted batch after batch in Maxwell's kitchen, combining oat bran, corn syrup, maltodextrin (a dry sweet thickener), milk protein, and peanut and sesame butters. Then they would field-test—Maxwell running and occasionally munching; Vaughan trailing him on a bicycle. Following that, they would shelf test by swaddling their creations in Saran wrap and dumping them on Maxwell's sunny dashboard. The results were not pretty. After a couple of weeks, the bars moldered, emitting an arresting barnyard perfume.

Vaughan, the science guy, came to the rescue. He had originally met Maxwell through a consulting gig at Protein Research, a company that develops and formulates nutritional supplements, and says of their relationship: "I was the chef and he was the cook." But while he had studied nutrition as part of his Ph.D. program, Vaughan was no food technologist. To solve the case of the odiferous confections, he turned to the Bioscience and Natural Resources Library at Berkeley, where a knowledgeable librarian, Norma Kobzina, who has since died, helped him find resources on controlling water activity. "Berkeley probably didn't subscribe to Food Science and Technology Abstracts [FSTA, an index that's the be-all and end-all of food technology research], but it would have been available through Dialog, and my guess is that Norma would have done a Dialog search," said Axel Borg, another career University of California librarian.

That search would have provided a road map on how to make moist and chewy food bars that could be stored at room temperature, part of the large body of scientific literature, most of it generated by academics, on which food companies rely to develop new products. If you do an FSTA search of water activity in moist foods between the years of 1970 and 1985, you get 101 results: articles, theses, conference proceedings, and patents. One author appears on more than one-seventh of these and on almost all the important ones—"The Effect of Water Activity on Reaction Kinetics of Food Deterioration," "Effect of Temperature on the Moisture Sorption Isotherms and Water Activity Shift of Two Dehydrated Foods," and "Prediction of Water Activity Lowering Ability of Food Humectants at High a_w"—Ted Labuza. There's nothing odd about that, of course. Every field has its experts; they get that way because their topics have intrinsic value, and the marketplace of ideas ensures that the cream rises to the top.

Vaughan now had the answer to his problem. He rejiggered the recipe, adding fructose to bind up more of the "free" water, bringing the water activity to below 0.85, which made the confection inhospitable to mold and the proteins in it less prone to enzymatic deterioration. He also dosed it with branched-chain amino acids, especially leucine, after reading an unpublished paper, "The Effects of Submaximal Exercise on Whole Body Leucine Metabolism," that found that endurance sports increased the consumption of this vital amino acid throughout the body. This became the first formulation for the PowerBar, which went into production in 1986. Buoyed by Brian's indefatigable appetite for racing—he was, in Vaughan's less than complimentary term, "a grinder"—and instinctive grasp of grassroots promotion, such as handouts at the local 10K, by 2000, the company's sales had ballooned to $150 million, the year it was sold to Nestlé for $375 million. Today the energy bar category is so crowded it commands its own shelf at the supermarket: Clif, Balance, LUNA, Atkins, and Odwalla are eagerly joined by the oldie-but-goodie conglomerates—primarily ready-to-eat cereal manufacturers, such as Kellogg's, Nature Valley (General Mills), and Nabisco.

It's a heartwarming tale: a couple of penniless but inspired entrepreneurs reenacting our favorite bootstrapping business origin story—the one that proves our meritocratic capitalistic system works, by gum. Their product, vindicated by multidigit sales growth, the result of old-fashioned American ingenuity—with maybe a kindly librarian thrown in for good measure.

Vaughan is vehement that the PowerBar has no military heritage and, in fact, rather testily characterizes army research as "pissing down a dark well." He continued to disavow any connection in response to several of my follow-up questions:

Did any of the scientific and technical resources he used have military origins?

"[The bioscience library] did not collect army/navy research documents. That would have been in the documents library, which was not a place to go to search for state-of-the-art nutritional information."

Was he aware of the Natick Center?

"Not in the least."

Did he know that the military had been researching food/energy bars since the early 1960s, including having had contracts with Pillsbury and General Foods to develop, among other things, cereal-based bars?

"Never heard of it."

How about intermediate-moisture foods?

"Never heard of it."*

Vaughan is not alone in his ignorance of the influence of military-funded or -orchestrated research on the very products he developed for the commercial market. Many food technologists don't even know what the Natick Center (or its predecessor organizations) is, let alone have an awareness of how it has steered the science and technology behind their industry. To understand its importance requires serious detective work. Identifying first-generation impacts—papers, patents, products—is hard enough, as credit is most often claimed by collaborators. But after that, the path to understanding why a particular scientific or technological direction was taken is long, circuitous, and dim, and must be cobbled together from article footnotes, long-ago meetings, professional relationships, and CVs. Unsurprisingly, military provenance often vanishes.

---

* In fact, even the PowerBar innovation of which Vaughan is most proud, the addition of leucine, the amino acid depleted during intense exercise, was based on military research. Work on the protein building block's role in metabolism was begun during the 1970s at the Letterman Army Institute of Research; the not-yet-published 1983 paper by several MIT and Tufts scientists Vaughan e-mailed me to demonstrate the "science behind the bar" was the outgrowth of a project done in part with Natick's U. S. Army Research Institute of Environmental Medicine.

Chapter 8

HOW DO YOU WANT THAT CHUNKED AND FORMED RESTRUCTURED STEAK?

LUNCH BOX ITEM #2: PACKAGED DELI MEAT

The ritual is unvarying. Around 6:00 p.m., I halt what I'm doing—reading 1940s chemical industry journals, making the umpteenth pass over a mumble in an interview, laboriously wringing out a sentence while steeling myself against the urge to check the news—and swing open the refrigerator door. I stand there for a long moment, staring, asking myself that eternal question, "What should I make for dinner?"

There are the traditional meals on the days I've had the foresight to set a package of frozen meat, poultry, or seafood to defrost in the morning: toaster-grilled marinated steak; shrimp sautéed with garlic, strips of lemon zest, and fresh thyme; *ajiaco bogateño,* a hearty Colombian chicken, caper, and potato stew. But more often than not, I stand there weighing the last-minute options: raid the freezer for a box of chicken or fish nuggets, patties, or cutlets, or hit the cheese drawer, which my husband keeps stocked with presliced hams, hot dogs, chicken sausages, and other prepared meats?

It's a choice that makes me uneasy, although it pleases my children, in whom I've failed to inculcate a taste for traditional animal flesh. But as the long ingredient list reveals, these bland, symmetrical substitutes are less healthy, maybe not healthy at all. When Jorge and I met, we discovered a startling coincidence: both of our fathers were statisticians. Later, our serious, upright fathers provided us with another: they both suddenly developed and died of pancreatic cancer. Jorge's father was a heavy smoker, a risk factor. But my dad, a runner, without an ounce of fat on him? I see him now, getting his lunch ready at bedtime so that when he left for work at 6:00 a.m. he could just slip into the darkness: two slapped-together sandwiches—bread, cheese, and packaged deli meat (turkey, ham, or roast beef). One of the few known risk factors for this most deadly cancer is a diet high in red and processed meat.[1] I push down the thought and reach for the hot dogs.

THE AMERICAN CARNIVORE—whether hypo, meso, or hyper in her habits—can go an entire week, month, or even year without confronting the animal origins of her favorite food. If she's hard-core, maybe the morning begins with bacon, once a hunk of pork belly but now an almost Art Deco assemblage of crispy, striped strips, or, something even further removed from its beginnings, the breakfast sausage. Lunch, whether packed in a brown paper bag from home or takeout from her favorite fast-food outlet, inevitably includes restructured protein, which quietly overtook all other forms of fauna-based products in the 1990s. Dinner is the closest she gets to the real deal—ground beef; boneless, skinless chicken breast; pork tenders.

Most people attribute the U.S. consumer's divorce from the realities of slaughtering, butchering, and preparing meat to a ridiculous squeamishness; we are chided for our reluctance to embrace the nose-to-tail gusto still prevalent in most of the world. (In this they are dead wrong: what, I ask you, is a better example of everything-but-the-squeal-or-moo than the humble hot dog?) This public relations jujitsu suits the powers that be just fine. The real reason for our apparent fondness for food made from refashioned animal tissue has nothing to do with our puerile taste buds—it has to do with the relentless quest by the U.S. Army to reduce the cost of the meat it uses to feed soldiers and, once it has found a way to do so, industry's giddy embrace of the same to lower the expense of producing, transporting, and storing the meat it sells you.

For centuries, having a bone in our dinner was an insurance policy. For those with a passing familiarity with the beasts, birds, and crawling creatures God so thoughtfully delivered into our dominion—a group that included everyone until well into the twentieth century—a length of calcium-fortified connective tissue was an indispensable feature for quick and easy identification of the animal and body part in question. It also made it that much harder for a butcher to disguise some of the disturbing things that can happen to meat—sickly source, decay, and forays by vermin. (Of course, these inroads didn't need to be an obstacle. An early nineteenth-century butchery how-to gives lessons in entomology, training *fleischmeisters* to distinguish no less than four species of flies, and provides this appetizing suggestion for dealing with *Musca*-egg-laden "blown meat": "The part should be taken out, and some pepper put upon the place.") Visual inspection happened both at the butcher stand or shop, where meat merchandising consisted of a spiked rack draped with gory carcasses and severed limbs, and at the table, where guests invited to dine with the local lords could be assured their dinner was of primo material by its appearance practically intact on a platter. The poor, in contrast, supped on the unrecognizable remnants of the brutes, mostly in stews and soups.

As in most passionate relationships, our feelings about meat are complicated. Nothing makes us feel quite like it does—the high protein content, the perfectly matched amino acids, the rich soup of elusive B vitamins and minerals. But it is also among the most fragile—and dangerous—of foodstuffs: if not brimming with spoilers and pathogens from the outset, then attracting and breeding a whole favela of unwelcome guests over time. Far worse, to partake of it, we must kill. Meat straddles the border between sacred and profane; every pork chop questions how much we value life; every hamburger reminds us of how frail it is. Is it any wonder the stuff makes us very, very nervous? This ambivalence extends to our societally sanctioned animal death professionals, butchers (as well as to the human ones, soldiers and executioners).

Our distaste for butchers and distrust of their wares wasn't helped by their work environments, which were traditionally a filthy mess. They were, in fact, a shambles, a word that originally meant butcher's digs. The occupational specialty appeared with the founding of cities, which, with their huddled masses, did not allow for the keeping of large grazing livestock (they did, however, allow for the small and garbage-consuming: backyard chickens and pigs were the original urbanites). The first butchers operated stands in open-air markets: farmers would arrive with their herds, most often goats and sheep but occasionally cattle, which would be slaughtered on the spot in a display of blood-spattering virtuosity. The gory by-products were left to fester in the already ordure-strewn street and ditches, giving rise to the sort of geographical nomenclature—Stinking Lane, Blowbladder Street—that discouraged company on daily errands.

Efforts to regulate the noisome trade, which by now was organized into powerful guilds—some butchers' guilds even had their own police forces—were regular and ongoing. Starting in the late fourteenth century, laws were passed banishing slaughter to outside city walls, mandating disposal of waste in pits, and forbidding the sale of "roten Schep"[2] and other sickly or rotting flesh. Slowly, the members of the Worshipful Company of Butchers began to move back downtown, transacting their business through large curved windows and finally, after it was invented in the 1800s, retreating behind plate glass (compressed air allowed glassmakers to partially cool large cylinders that could then be sliced opened and flattened). The only public evidence of their guilt-inducing activities was the rack hung with artfully composed swags made from their victims' bodies, a practice that was finally expunged toward the end of the nineteenth century, when cities and towns got to work sanitizing the streetscape. Still, the old hierarchy of cuts based on proximity to the bone remained, with the best being the primals and the worst the odds and ends left behind after all the cutting was done.

Meat, or rather the muscles from which it comes, defines us and the taxonomic kingdom to which we belong, Animalia. Its name is derived from the Latin word for the huffing and puffing done by its members, which, at least in mammals, is powered by the diaphragm, a round, flat muscle that buckles back and forth creating air flow by continually changing the volume of the lungs. Cardiac fibers play percussion through the long days of our (hopefully) long lives. Smooth muscles push blood, lymph, food, urine, excrement, semen, and babies through the various channels, chutes, tubes, and tunnels that riddle our bodies. But it is the skeletal muscles lining our bones and padding our forms that truly liberate us. Able to go wherever and do whatever we please, we animals, more than any other beings in the great tree of life, are the agents of our own destinies.

There are two basic kinds of muscle cells. Fast-twitch or white fibers specialize in quick movements—lunges, darts, jabs, and feints; they are run on casual hookups with stored or blood glucose and, like most sugar addicts, rapidly need another fix. Slow-twitch or red fibers are long-haul plodders; their metabolic relationships are much more serious. Myoglobin, an overdeveloped molecular bodyguard composed of more than 150 amino acids, escorts an oxygen molecule from the blood to the mitochondria, private chambers where, in a really, really long chain reaction, the cell combusts it with fat. The souped-up security is for a reason: oxygen and fat produce thirty-six energy-giving ATP molecules compared with sugar's measly two.

Of course, all the intricate cellular machinery goes straight to hell once an animal's heart has been stopped and its body hacked into pieces. After oxygen transportation ceases, the mitochondria are shuttered for good, leaving the slam-bam-thank-you-ma'am enzymes to wander disconsolately, gobbling up any remaining sugar—and excreting lactic acid, which slowly lowers the pH and imparts a slightly sour, though not unpleasant, taste to the flesh. When the energy-generating enzymes have sputtered to a stop, the muscle fibers, without ATP to release them, are mortared together by calcium and left in one final, agonized contraction: rigor mortis has set in.

At that point, enzymes that break apart proteins, including calpains, begin to dismantle the muscle's structural elements—ligaments, tendons, cartilage, and tension-maintaining elastin. (The harder a muscle works, the more connective tissue it has; one of the tenderest muscles of any animal is the lazy longissimus, which runs along the spine and whose only job is to keep it straight.) Later, when the pH is lower still, the reinforcements arrive, including cathepsins, acid-loving enzymes housed in a special organelle now burst open by the low pH. These enzymes tenderize the meat, a process that requires about a day for poultry, a week for pork, and anywhere from two weeks to a month for beef. The different aging rates may be because fast-twitch fibers have a higher proportion of stored glucose, so tend to go through the chemical breakdown faster than slow-twitch fibers, as well as offer a better-supplied larder to marauding decomposers.

The usual suspects are most often several varieties of *Pseudomonas,* a hearty little spoilage bacterium that thrives equally well not only in cold and warm temperatures but also in acid, neutral, and alkaline environments. It is happy to dine on whatever happens to be available, although glucose is always its first choice. When that's exhausted, *Pseudomonas* keeps on digging, downing debris from amino acids for its energy source. Unfortunately, the digestion of these can engender noxious fumes, as anyone who has ordered the eighteen-ounce porterhouse at Sizzler can vouch, due to their breakdown into the malodorous amines. Our raw pork chop starts to stink.

Until the mid-nineteenth century, locally raised and slaughtered fresh meat wasn't a nicety—it was a necessity. Long-distance transport of unpreserved animal flesh was potentially lethal for the end user. There was an exception: since time immemorial, humankind has known that cold delays decay, even without knowing why (it makes the bacteria that share our taste in comestibles very, very sluggish). For this reason, unless sacrificing the requisite ruminant or monogastric for a feast, the eating of fresh meat had always been a seasonal activity in temperate zones. Slaughter was done during early winter, and the carcass divested of its drapery in the frigid months that followed. Once the earth's axis pointed toward the sun again, however, January's gifts disappeared, except for occasional pockets left in caves or root cellars.

In the early nineteenth century, the renegade son of a prominent Boston family, Frederic Tudor, teamed up with a Cambridge, Massachusetts, townie, Nathaniel Wyeth, to found one of the most lucrative industries of the time: frozen water. Using Wyeth's invention, blades strapped on a plow, they carved up winter lakes into blocks, stacked the blocks with sawdust mortar in special icehouses and insulated ship holds, and sent them from New England to the south and the Caribbean. The ships' crews quickly noticed the cargo's ability to keep tipples and nibbles chilled en route, and the concept of the cold chain was born. By the 1870s, ice-cooled reefers, the industry term for refrigerated cargo ships, were making their maiden voyages carrying "dead meat." Within the next quarter century, consumer and commercial demand—particularly in the meat-packing, dairy, and brewing trades—for solid-state H_2O mushroomed, as did fortunes founded on the stuff. Later, the ice was swapped for modern refrigeration machines rigged together from compressors, condensers, coils, and coolants made of volatile, and flammable, chemicals. By 1905 millions of globe-trotting beef quarters from Argentina, Australia, New Zealand, and the United States were crisscrossing the Atlantic in freighters kept cold by an ammonia solution (the principal ingredient was made from dung- and guano-based nitrate, an ingredient in gunpowder) that was put through its phase-changing paces—first a vapor, then a liquid, again a vapor, again a liquid—alternately absorbing and dumping excess heat.

★ ★ ★

THE SINGLE MOST EXPENSIVE ITEM on the military menu has always been meat, generally accounting for more than half the bill. For starters, as most vegetarians, animal activists, and environmentalists have pointed out at one time or another, animal flesh takes a flabbergasting amount of land, water, and plant food to produce. "Harvesting" it is a full-scale event, until the twentieth century requiring the labor of highly trained professionals, as is processing the "crop" into edible group- or individual-size portions. And finally, because meat is so alluring to itsy-bitsy life-forms, and so biologically complex that even after death it undergoes all sorts of still little-understood changes, it must be stored and transported with great care—and expense.

During the Civil War, the flesh in the regulation tin bowls of the 2.1 million Union army recruits arrived the old-fashioned way, "on the hoof," a transportation method that had its demerits. Some animals inconsiderately died en route. Others took the opportunity to crash-diet, losing up to sixty pounds during the trek. All had the inconvenient habit of requiring large amounts of water and forage along the way. By the Spanish-American War in 1898, refrigerated railcars and steamship holds enabled the shipping of carcasses, which, for a force of about 300,000 men, didn't unduly tax the infrastructure. But when the United States reluctantly joined World War I in 1917, it faced a more than tenfold increase in the demand for chow. How to keep 4.7 million recruits in their promised pound o' protein a day? Suddenly the lifestyle to which future tenderloins had grown accustomed—ceiling hooks in a refrigerated hold placed so they could swing, jiggle, and sway without disturbing their similarly situated neighbors—was too luxurious. Desperate to keep supplies running, the U.S. Army Quartermaster Corps, led by Chief of Subsistence Colonel William Grove, put on its thinking cap: Could it go against humankind's age-old antipathy to barrels of unidentifiable chunks and scraps, long disdained as containing tainted meat? Could we send our boys boneless beef?

In 1918, under the expansionist eye of Lieutenant Jay Hormel, the army set up the very first boxed-beef processing plant and distribution system, centered in Chicago. The results caused army bigwigs to do a little jig: a quarter carcass weighed 25 percent less without its bones, fat, and cartilage and, when frozen into a rectangular solid, wrapped in burlap and waxed paper, and stacked, occupied 60 percent less space on crowded trains and ships. Soon hundred-pound boxes were shipping out to France; in all, about 8 percent of the 449 million pounds of beef consumed during the war arrived this way. There were, however, a few kinks. It turns out that dumping everything together and freezing it created a god-awful mess. Individual cuts were difficult to thaw, which engendered mutinous mess hall grumbling—how come he gets a porterhouse and I get a burger?—and just plain didn't look good (slowly freezing meat busts open its cells and intracellular structures, turning its surface dark brown). Army cooks took to hacking the blocks apart with axes, resulting in, as the official historians tactfully put it, "unattractive and often unpalatable" fare.

The first attempt at a boneless beef product hadn't gone very well, but the army is nothing if not persistent. Based in Chicago, where the Big Five meatpackers—Armour, Swift, Morris, Wilson, and Cudahy— were located, the Quartermaster Corps Subsistence School (and, after 1936, its descendant, the Subsistence Research Laboratory) plugged away at the problem during the 1920s and 1930s. But they didn't make progress until Jesse White from the Navy Veterinary Department, who spearheaded the project, enlisted the help of Armour and Swift in 1938. A new boning technique was developed that got almost all the edible meat off the carcass. Meat was sorted into different classes instead of a single frozen block of undifferentiated animal parts: each container held packages of roasts and steaks (40 percent), chunks for soups and stews (30 percent), and—don't look too closely—grinding grade (30 percent). Additionally, rather than deep-freeze the box of meat and let the cold penetrate the flesh over hours or days, they flash froze it. (The frozen boxes could also be used to keep other perishables cool.) The technique, which uses extremely low temperatures, was invented by Clarence Birdseye, the "father" of frozen food; the method doesn't rupture cell walls and produces smaller ice crystals, resulting in meat or plant tissue that's almost like fresh in appearance and texture.

The Quartermaster Corps' innovations came just in time for the Greatest Generation, who laced up their boots and tromped off across the continents, while their Rosies riveted fighter planes and grew victory gardens. By the end of World War II, there were casualties on an unimaginable scale—the United States alone lost almost 400,000 troops. Although not generally recognized, the humble American cow also made staggering sacrifices: 29 million gave their lives to feed enlisted men and women from 1941 to 1945. They arrived to overseas battle theaters boneless, frozen, and boxed. This preparation cut in half the number of cargo ships needed to navigate hostile waters and allowed an irregularly shaped product to be neatly piled and palletized (fastened to a flat carrier), an innovation that didn't originate with the military but got a critical bump in its dissemination by the war.

But that was just the beginning. Boxed boneless beef offered a whole panoply of value-added propositions that the army magnanimously bestowed on its associates in the meatpacking industry—they could charge more, because the product required additional time and labor, and they could keep and sell the hides (leather), fat (soap and margarine), bones (stock, fertilizer, and tankage, or protein supplements for animal feed), and trimmings. (It's probably no coincidence that the first packaged hot dog—Oscar Mayer's Kartridg-Pak, a product later encased in Saran—appeared in Chicago at about the same time.) For the military, the new product also had additional benefits. Cooking and serving the new cuts took fewer personnel and less time, leaving more leisure for important things like gossiping and ribbing your fellow soldiers, who were in a much better mood now that dining didn't involve dueling for T-bones. And, joy of joys, the streamlined slices of meat eliminated the smelly piles of viscera that had for eons added a down-market vibe to the mess hall landscaping. The Defense Department, convinced it had a hit on its hands, crowed, "Military advances in beef processing have made the beef ration a reality almost everywhere that our present global Army may be. The Army has put boneless beef—frozen fresh and packed so that there can be no mistakes in cooking and serving—on a basis where further experimentation is not necessary. It is now ready for civilian use."[3]

Not quite.

It turned out American housewives had their own ideas about how fresh meat should be sold, and it didn't involve removing the internal scaffolding or subjecting it to temperatures below 32°F. Earnest attempts in the late 1940s and 1950s by Chicago meatpackers, already rubbing their hands over visions of fortunes to be made with the new more convenient meats, were a bust. Swift, which had helped develop and then supplied the military with frozen boxed beef during World War II, produced a frozen rectangular roast that flopped. At a special 1959 conference on the future of beef, sponsored by the National Academy of Sciences–National Research Council, advertising executives, the food industry, agricultural businesses, and academia mulled over how to persuade the recalcitrant consumer to accept boneless beef, even if it was, by their own estimation, inferior: "Tastes can be changed. This is [a challenge] . . . you have to face, particularly as we enter into the area of consumer convenience foods, because obviously here you have to make certain kinds of compromises to prepare these products."

It took almost fifty years, and happened in phases, but over time the economic and practical benefits of boxed boneless meat (sometimes frozen and sometimes even seasoned—hello, Trader Joe's) were too great to ignore. By the 1960s the former Big Four meatpackers (two merged), weakened by the government's 1948 antitrust attacks on their vertically integrated business model (own the stockyards, own the packinghouse, own the railroad, own the truck, own the storage depot, own the wholesale center) as well as the inadequacy of that model for the postwar era, had been acquired, merged, or gone out of business. A new Big Four—Iowa Beef Packers, now Iowa Beef Processors (IBP); Cargill; Tyson Foods; and JBS (together responsible for 85 percent of all beef slaughter in 2010)—arose phoenixlike to take their place. Chief among these was IBP, which had put into practice several innovative (and cost-saving) ideas: buy cheap real estate near large feedlots and set up shop there (the federal highway system freed them from the railroads); jettison the old-guard system of hooks, tables, and skilled butchers and institute one of conveyor belts and low-skilled labor with a few simple tasks to do as the carcass drifted by; and, most important, do the final "boning and breaking" of the animal into retail cuts on-site, which meant they could sell boxes full of a single item, be it choice rib-eye steaks, select boneless rounds, chuck, or ungraded ground beef.

This time the lady of the house—and, yes, most groceries were, and still are, bought by women—was in the mood. In fact, what with her Frigidaire and new job as a typist, she was verging on desperate for quick ways to get dinner on the table. Between 1963 and 2002, the percentage of boxed beef shipped from the nation's largest slaughter houses increased from less than 10 percent to 60 percent of their total sales, and now accounts for more than 90 percent of the beef sold in supermarkets.

In the modestly titled *Iowa Beef Processors, Inc.: An Entire Industry Revolutionized!*, the former IBP president Dale Tinstman lays stake to the breakthrough idea behind their success: "It was a natural progression from the efficiencies of shipping carcasses to shipping boxed beef. There is a lot of wasted space in a modern truck or rail car filled with chilled sides of beef. A side of beef has an awkward shape—it can't be neatly packed, and a side has a lot of bone and trim that will never go into the meat case. It was logical to move to boxed beef."

Nary a word about the ossa-free meat he surely refueled on during his days of navigating B-29 bombers during World War II, or saw riffling through *Life* magazine in the mid-1940s, where full-page ads by the American Meat Institute trumpeted boxed boneless meat developed for the U.S. Army Quartermaster Corps as one of its industry's "most noteworthy war developments."

★ ★ ★

TO PARAPHRASE JFK PARAPHRASING MUSSOLINI'S SON-IN-LAW, failure is an orphan, but success has a thousand fathers. These are usually smiling jovially as they viciously elbow one another out of the family photo. Such is the case of McDonald's (in)famous McRib, a washboard-shaped cutlet composed of porcine oddments, soaked in treacly barbecue sauce, strewn with pickles and onions, and stuffed in an oblong bun.

The iconic sandwich debuted in 1981 in sixty-five stores in six cities as a way to contain costs during a recession when overall sales were slack. "McDonald's is 'doing the best we can' to keep from raising prices, a company spokesman says," reported the *Christian Science Monitor*. At first interest was so low, the fast-food company gave the item away for breakfast; even then, "consumers simply turned up their noses," but eventually (a good twenty years later), the pig meat–stuffed roll became a hit. Appreciation may have been fanned by scarcity; in the early days, the pork product appeared and disappeared several times from the McDonald's menu, and is now only available for a short time once a year in the United States. By the early aughts, promoted by social media frenzies worth their weight in broadcast media buys, the McRib had gained a permanent foothold in the market and an ardent following. And suddenly everyone claimed to have invented it.

We can quickly eliminate contender #1, Rene Arend, McDonald's French-trained chief chef, whose inspiration was the ersatz baby back shape and secret spices and toppings. But delve deeper than the finishing flourishes to the actual process for creating the restructured pork patty, and the story gets complicated—and competitive.

Contender #2, Dr. Roger Mandigo, an academic eager beaver, a Meat Industry Hall of Famer, and a professor emeritus from the University of Nebraska, says the following:

> In about 1970 we started working on restructured meat. . . . It came about because the National Pork Council was looking for ways to get more pork into fast-food menus. We proposed the idea of restructuring pork; it could be in any shape or form. The project was funded by the National Pork Council with the pork producers' check-off fund—a nickel for every hog. . . . Our original restructured pork was shaped like chops; McDonald's adapted them for their McRibs.

Or perhaps we should credit contender #3, Dr. Dale Huffman, a laid-back and low-key researcher, famous for his 91 percent fat-free burger, retired from a forty-year stint at Alabama's Auburn University?

> The genesis goes back to my one-year industrial fellowship at Armour in 1969–70. I had interaction with people there who were making a restructured product, flaked and formed, which was good, but it didn't have the characteristics of a muscle meat. When I got back to the university, Bettcher [a food- and meat-processing equipment company in Ohio] made equipment available which we moved into our pilot plant at Auburn University. Our greatest success was with the pork chop. [Joe Cordray, my partner, and I] took a truckload of product to [the] National Pork Council annual meeting in St. Louis. . . . Burger King was interested in using our

restructured pork chop, but the parent company in Great Britain vetoed it. The only product in the marketplace today that you can trace back is the McDonald's McRib.

But wait. Another candidate has appeared. Now retired, contender #4, John Secrist, a humble but devoted food technologist at the Natick Soldier Research, Development and Engineering Center, once turned down a promotion so he could spend more time in the lab.

> The Armed Forces Product Evaluation Committee asked us what we could do to reduce the price of steaks and chops and things like that. . . . So we started a flaking project with this company from Ohio, Bettcher Industries, which was interested in getting more business from their flaking machines. . . . We could make it look like anything—pork chops, lamb chops. . . . Almost all of the meatpackers did trial production runs for us at no cost because . . . if it was satisfactory to the military, they'd leapfrog over the rest of the industry because they'd be the ones who did it first. Denny's used our restructured beefsteak in their restaurant; still do. And McDonald's McRib is as close to our product as you can get.

Americans have always taken pride in the fact that military messes served nothing but the finest to our boys and girls in uniform. After all, the mostly young Americans who risk their lives defending our country deserve that delicious, nutritious, ne plus ultra of warrior foods: meat. Pink and unctuous steak, seared and steaming chops, hearty stews, grill-charred patties, all cut from choice nine-hundred-pound steers. That ideal changed in the 1960s, when supermarkets finally saw the light and embraced the armed forces' world-war innovation of butchering, sorting, and packaging beef at the point of slaughter. The growing demand for boxed beef tipped the balance away from carcass beef, and meatpackers, through their advocacy organization, the American Meat Institute, let it be known that Uncle Sam better get with its new program and buy its meat by cut and grade like everybody else. (Until then, because it purchased in such large quantities at relatively short notice, the army had bought whole carcasses.)

It was a golden opportunity. Now, thanks to the military's mammoth purchasing power, it could finally upgrade the offering, negotiating rock-bottom prices for millions of pounds of steak and standing ribs. Top brass considered the possibility for a millisecond and then they shook their heads. "Now that we can finally buy just the cuts we want, how about we get the cheapest stuff there is and figure out a way to get the grunts to eat it?" Armed forces executives set the goal of reducing the meat bill by 60 percent with the as-yet undiscovered way to turn a sow's ear into a cute little pork steakette. The challenge was on.

Natick Center food scientists went into the laboratory and began to fiddle, as well as to contract with universities and industry for outside research. There was, after all, a long history of turning trimmings and less desirable cuts into something tasty—*la charcuterie,* or, in good old American English, cold cuts. Four basic techniques, in use for centuries in practically every place people partake of animal flesh, went into making these foodstuffs: chopping or grinding, binding, shaping, and, finally, cooking or curing. The difference between humankind's mouthwatering grab bag of salami, sausage, bologna, and frankfurters and what the Natick Center was doing was one of intent: traditional meat products don't pretend to be anything but what they are, a scraps-to-scrumptious redemption story. The army's invention, on the other hand, was meant to fool; the closer scientists got to getting your eye, nose, tongue, and teeth to believe their creation was the real thing, the happier they were.

It wasn't easy. And it didn't happen in one big eureka moment, but in piecing together a series of discoveries that occurred over a decade or so. The first, in a late 1950s patent assigned to Oscar Mayer—by then one of the nation's largest and most successful meat products companies—was that tumbling or massaging large chunks of meat with salt caused them to ooze a sticky fluid that, upon cooking, would cohere them. The second significant advance came from equipment suppliers. During the early 1960s, Bettcher Industries of Ohio, came up with a new design for a flaking machine. Instead of pushing the meat against a guillotine, a process that also squeezed out the water, a circular head spun it toward fixed blades on the perimeter. This shaved the meat paper-thin, maximizing surface area while conserving the juices. Third, a new understanding of how muscles work in living and dead animals allowed food technologists to begin to manipulate and control these processes. Using the electron microscope, scientists observed that muscle fibers are composed of smaller fibers called myofibrils, which in turn are composed of strands of the proteins myosin and actin. By momentarily binding together in a sort of rowing motion, these two proteins contract the muscle. They ooze out of the ruptured meat cells and, under the conditions described in the Oscar Mayer patent, dissolve into the surrounding fluid to create a "meat glue." The final important finding—by Natick researchers in the early 1970s—was that adding a small amount of phosphate to the salt shifted the pH of the meat, which allowed its molecules to spread out and retain more water, improving juiciness, texture, and flavor.

By the mid-1960s, army scientists working on the restructured meat project were giving glowing internal reports to higher-ups. In a 1966 presentation, Natick food technologists announced that they had developed a "highly acceptable fabricated 'beef steak' which is among the meat items heat stabilized in flexible pouches. This 'steak' is prepared by a proprietary process involving adding a small amount of salt to trimmings, treating in a manner to cover all surfaces with heat coagulatable protein, pressing into a mold or casing, heating to a temperature sufficient to 'set' the protein, and eventually cutting to serving size. . . . The process is presumably applicable to pork, veal and poultry." The Advisory Board on Military Personnel Supplies' subcommittee on meat products all but jumped up and down with enthusiasm, proclaiming in italics: "*The future of fabricated modules of meat [is] excellent and that studies in this area should be continued.*" By 1972 the army's fake-muscle-cuts project had progressed sufficiently to contract out several pilot production runs, including mechanically formed grill steaks, Swiss steaks, minute steaks, and breakfast steaks. It started serving the troops restructured veal cutlets in 1976, followed by lamb and pork chops, and, somewhat later, beefsteaks. The idea had legs. Speculated a 1980 *New York Times* News Service article about the Natick Center invention, "Restructured meats could trim the food budget for the average consumer as well since these products may become increasingly available in restaurants, cafeterias and the frozen foods departments of supermarkets all over the country." Such as, say, McDonald's.

By the early 1980s, the military's role in developing and promoting interest in restructured meat was winding down. The private sector's, on the other hand, was ramping up, its appetite whetted by the value-added proposition of making something from practically nothing. University and industry food-science departments soon found ways to further reduce manufacturing costs by stripping every little last bit of protein from carcasses, including hot deboning (you got it: while the corpse is still steaming), desinewing, mechanical separation (pushing a carcass through a sieve), blending fat and trim into protein "sludge," and collection of plasma for use as a plumper. To expand the product line from the frozen foods section to the refrigerator case, new binders that didn't require heat to set were created in a variety of fun flavors, such as cow's blood and pig's blood clotting factor, bacterial enzymes, algae, and chemicals. Consumption of restructured meat products exploded during the 1990s and early years of the 2000s—so much so that in 1997 the Census Bureau had to add a new industry code. That year, (nonpoultry) meat processing, which manufactures products, generated $2.4 billion in sales, almost half of the $5.4 billion generated by the meatpacking industry itself, which slaughters, butchers, and distributes. By 2007 processing accounted for $3.7 billion and meatpacking $6.9 billion— together an astounding $10.6 billion in flesh-prep sales. Is it any surprise that by the twenty-first century Americans were eating more animal protein than ever before—close to 200 pounds, up from about 140 pounds in 1950?

The public, however, didn't seem to notice the sea change in its eating habits—entranced as it was by blogging and tweeting about the cyclical appearance and disappearance of its new favorite fast food, the threescore and ten–ingredient McRib (the item is only available when pork trim is affordable). Journalists, ever eager to put a human face on a story, dubbed Professor Mandigo—who, although he did not bring this up during our interview, contracted his services to Natick on other meat projects—the proud father not only of the McRib but, almost as an after-thought, of restructured meat, and while he's careful not to make this claim himself, he's never disavowed it either. At least until now. When I asked him point-blank if the U.S. Army had come up with the concept, he hemmed and hawed, then mumbled, "Natick's influence was through the literature and through technology transfer. Government doesn't patent their intellectual property, so anyone can use it. They presented material at technical meetings. People would say, I can use that, but had slight variations on the technology. The military allowed us to use the processes they'd developed."

Exactly.

It took the U.S. Army almost a century to pry the bone-in steak from the public grip, but now our feelings about meat are reversed. Embold-ened by science (microbiology) and technology (refrigeration), we no longer demand bodily evidence as to the origins and wholesomeness of our dinner and have even learned to prefer our animal in the forms pioneered by the military: boneless, which halves its shipping volume, and restructured, which allows cheaper cuts to be substituted for more expensive ones. By far most of the animal protein we eat has been reas-sembled from bits and pieces by machines and is purchased everywhere but the meat department—deli case, frozen foods section, vending machine, cafeteria, drive-through. Only on rare occasions do we approach the gleaming counter with its ruby jewels of flesh. The once almighty butcher is now just a jocular salesperson whose job it is to weigh, wrap, and spout cooking tips. The magnificent crown of lamb, the burly standing rib, the succulent pork leg, with their osseous flourishes, have been relegated to ceremonial occasions—Passover, Easter, or birth-days ending in zero—when we light candles, gather around the table, and remember, ever so fleetingly, our fraught and violent relationship to the rest of the animal world.

Chapter 9

A LOAF OF EXTENDED-LIFE BREAD, A HUNK OF PROCESSED CHEESE, AND THOU

LUNCH BOX ITEMS #3, #4, AND #5: SLICED BREAD, PROCESSED CHEESE, AND CHEESY CRACKERS

The only time I've truly enjoyed bread was during the four years I lived in Ecuador in the 1990s. My future husband and I bought baguettes daily at the *panadería* near our apartment. Every morning we took turns slicing them lengthwise, spreading the pieces (me, sloppily; him, carefully) with a locally made American-style peanut butter (my taste of home) and *mermelada de guayaba* (his), and serving it to the other in bed with *café con leche.* It left our mattress on the floor full of crumbs, but it tasted heavenly—sweet, gooey, and crunchy—and was so satisfying that neither of us would eat again until we met for *almuerzo,* hearty lunch, or at home after a long day of editing (me, in English; him, in Spanish).

But that was just an interlude. My primary relationship, like that of most Americans, has been with the spongy white or wheat slices stacked in a twist tie–closed plastic bag. They've been there for as long as I can remember—or rather, can't remember, for aside from my maternal grand-mother's almost blackened, buttery toast and the limp, American cheese sandwiches my mother made for car trips, I can barely bring into focus the bread from my childhood. Those same whole wheat, twelve-grain, oatmeal, or white loaves are now the staple in our house, residing in a wood-lined, aluminum 1950s bread box. The contents of the packages never seem to stale—although they occasionally mold after a couple of weeks—just dwindle to a pair of sad-sack heels. In the almost two decades we've been raising children, I've never seen any family member grab a piece and just eat it, whether for pleasure or hunger. And I certainly can't imagine a young couple, both alone and far from home, turning the square slices into silent declarations of love. Today our bread is most noticeable when absent. "Could you pick up a loaf when you're at the market?"

WHETHER BREAD HAS BEEN A NET GAIN OR LOSS for humanity is open to debate; that it has been a boon for dentistry is not. Ever since sinking our teeth into the first loaf—pounded, macerated emmer seeds, a type of early wheat, mixed with water and baked—our oral health has gone downhill. Egyptians, who invented the foodstuff, had the worst teeth ever: ground to stumps by debris-laden, artisanally milled grains; pocked with cavities from bacterial infestation; and marked by deep abscesses, often to the bone, from gum disease. Nonetheless, the North Africans loved their carbs, and with more than forty different types, were never at a loss for their daily—or hourly—bread.

Like those of other ancient civilizations, early Egyptian baked goods were a testament to man's desperation to make something palatable from the unremitting monotony of a grain-based diet. Still, after all that tiresome Little Red Hen activity (planting, tending, harvesting, threshing, grinding, mixing, and cooking), the result was flat and tough. It would take the accidental discovery of yeast to turn the foodstuff from frumpy to fabulous. Many food archaeologists believe that the uplifting impact of the microbes might have been discovered when a bowl of mash was left to sit overnight, but equally likely, given our propensity for partying, is that its origin was linked to the preparation of bread's naughty fraternal twin, beer.

Thus was born the protobaguette. The leavened loaf, the original convenience food—no pots, no plates, and no utensils needed—debuted about six thousand years ago. Wheat flour, for which today we use red, white, and hard varieties rather than antiquity's less pliable emmer, has unique properties stemming from its extraspecial protein, the much-maligned gluten. (Celiac disease affects an estimated 2 percent of the population. It may have been a human adaptation to maximize host nutrition from cereal foods while infested with worms.)[1] Gluten macromolecules—of which one of their components, glutenin, is nature's largest protein—when mixed and kneaded, begin to snag on one another and form lengthy, cross-linked chains. The protein strands are studded with starch molecules, long, branched spirals with a hollow at the center, which easily absorb water, becoming a viscous gel. Gluten gives bread its sponginess; starch, its silkiness. But all this would be just a bland, leaden mass if it weren't for effervescent yeast.

Yeast, like many of its microbial brethren, is a switch-hitter, changing metabolic pathways at the drop of a hat. There's the efficient but cumbersome aerobic pathway, supplying a hefty payload of thirty-one energy-giving ATP molecules, which occurs when there's plenty of oxygen and food, sugar or its sumo-weight cousin starch. Both the sugar and starch molecules are built of the same basic unit, a chain or ring of carbon festooned with oxygen and hydrogen, but sugar is the size equivalent of a single-family home, while starch can be anything from a large apartment complex to a good-size city. The by-product of this route is—bubble, bubble, bubble—carbon dioxide and water. And then there's the less-efficient but quick 'n' easy anaerobic pathway, delivering only two ATP, which occurs in oxygen-limited environments again with an ample food source; its by-products are fizzy carbon dioxide and ethanol.

The latter pathway, called fermentation, has proved so valuable to us that it's been the motive for the capture and forced labor of a particularly sweet-toothed yeast species, *Saccharomyces cerevisiae*. A classic sycophant, *S. cerevisiae* is all smiles with its master (us) and a ruthless killer with its microbe peers, using aerobic metabolism to reproduce rapidly, crowding out competitors, and anaerobic metabolism to poison them with toxic levels (to other microorganisms, not to us—at least in moderation) of its waste, alcohol. In beer, both by-products remain in the liquid, while in bread, the hooch is removed, first by venting the dough with a punch and then through evaporation during cooking. Of course, this dominance strategy is double-edged. Once the alcohol level has reached a certain percentage, it kills the yeast itself.

Although tradesmen initially had no clue how fermentation worked—was it magic, spontaneous generation, or something in the air?—for centuries breweries and bakeries had a symbiotic relationship based on their essential ingredient, with the bread makers exchanging cash for used mash to employ as starter. Meanwhile, while not exactly closing in on the cause, beer makers and scientists got a lot better at separating the element that was causing all the hubbub. In the late 1600s, Antoni van Leeuwenhoek vastly improved the microscope, a magnifying glass used in his day job as a cloth merchant to inspect fabric, by figuring out how to make very small glass spheres that could then be ground into powerful lenses. (This paved the way for the development of the modern compound microscope.) With these, he was able to spy on the doings of bacteria and protozoa—stunning the world with the news that there were "animalcules" all around us—as well as to see tiny inert spheres (yeast) in beer. In 1838 Charles Cagniard de la Tour, a French baron and tireless dabbler, postulated that yeast might be a plant after observing reproduction by budding and carbon dioxide bubbles. But until Louis Pasteur—whom you can also thank for the principles of food sterilization and vaccination—showed conclusively in 1858 that fermentation was accomplished through these tiny balls, that they were alive, and that oxygen accelerated their growth but inhibited fermentation, yeast manufacturing didn't really take off.

As is par for the course with us humans, it wasn't for an entirely high-minded reason. An improved continuous whisky still, patented in 1830, had been invented by Aeneas Coffey (an Irishman, of course). Distillation works because alcohol has a lower boiling point than water.

When you heat a liquid composed of both to 173°F, the alcohol boils out and can be captured as vapor. But a mixture of liquids behaves as a system, altering the boiling point for all, so this vapor contains quite a bit of water. In a continuous still, the vapor travels through a series of chambers at progressively lower temperatures, removing more water at every step. The new invention ran tubing through not one but two high columns, eliminating the need for a midprocess transfer of the liquid and upping the potency of the final product. Suddenly it was possible to make a tidy profit by dumping industrially produced yeast into a mash of cheap grain (or even tubers; hats off to the vodka belt of eastern Europe).

Within a few years, Jacques van Marken founded the first "yeast and methylated spirits" factory in Delft, the Netherlands, and the Fleischmann brothers set up an eponymous compressed-yeast-and-gin operation in Cincinnati, Ohio. These days, you can still find the cheery yellow-and-red packets in the baking aisle and the slightly seedy-looking bottle—the brand is not high on the price-point scale—at the liquor store. Both Fleischmann businesses prospered, and rivals such as Red Star, which began as Meadow Springs Distillery in 1882—almost always linking bread and booze—were founded. By the early twentieth century, most bakers relied on commercial starters obtained from yeast makers/distillers, which were now sold in damp, centrifuged cakes. The live yeast didn't travel well, however, perishing within ten days even when refrigerated. If companies wanted to expand their market areas, they had to build local production centers. By the early 1940s, Fleischmann's had seven plants in the continental United States, two in Canada, and three in Latin America. (Rotgut gin, of course, is perfectly fine at room temperature and needed no such pampering.)

The clunky regional yeast distribution system may have worked all right during peacetime, but it was woefully inadequate for World War I soldiers, who expected a daily sixteen-ounce ration of fresh white "American" bread—supplied by a special Quartermaster Corps bakery company—with their meals when stationed abroad. This problem turned into a full-fledged nightmare during World War II, with its unprecedented number of enlisted men and women to feed (not to mention the occasional "untimely appearance of shell fragments in the dough").[2] Shipping live compressed yeast to all corners of the globe was nigh impossible; local supplies were sometimes nonexistent or hard to come by—in Europe, for example, the Italians, Belgians, and Luxembourgers shared their stores, but the French, hoarding for their beloved baguettes, at first balked. It was time for the Subsistence Research Laboratory to work miracles by figuring out how to induce a state of suspended animation that could be easily lifted by bakers half a world away, months into the future, and in extreme climatic conditions.

The goal was to dry out the yeast but preserve all of its essential structures—cell wall, organelles, DNA/RNA, and enzymes—so that later it could be rehydrated and put to work. A few companies, notably Northwestern Yeast Company, did manufacture dried yeast, but it took almost a day to activate and didn't have the six- to eight-month shelf life required by the army. Fleischmann's, of course, was asked to work on the problem, as were other yeast companies, such as Red Star Yeast (the brand is now owned by Lesaffre Yeast Corporation and Archer Daniels Midland), and universities. Because there were no theories as to what might induce boundless hebetude in the microbes, the researchers followed the hallowed "cook and look" protocol, fooling around until something worked. "It will not be possible to describe the vast numbers of experiments that were tried," noted the Quartermaster Corps in a publication on the topic a decade later.[3] Different strains of the fungus were tested out. Variables were changed—more heat, less time; less time, more heat. Even the army's sensation du jour, freeze-drying, was given a whirl; the only thing it succeeded at was an 80 percent kill rate. Eventually, they hit upon the answer: grow the yeast in a relatively nitrogen-poor environment, extrude it in "spaghetti" strips, and then expose it to a stream of warm, dry air for six to eight hours, which reduces its moisture content to 8 percent (that of the compressed cakes was 70 percent).

It would take another forty years before scientists would understand why this worked. The secret was a substance called trehalose, a sugar molecule—experiments at the time found yeast to contain up to 18 percent trehalose. It had been assumed that trehalose was another carbohydrate storage molecule, but in the late 1980s scientists began to elucidate a protective function. Under environmental stress, yeast (and many other organisms) increases trehalose production, especially around the cell membrane where water molecules attach to it like an insulating layer. This allows it to stay limber despite heat, cold, drying, and other insults. Active dry yeast stored in foil packets—their inhabitants' long dormancy sheltered by trehalose—was supplied to garrison and field kitchens from 1944 until Victory Day in 1945, bringing the homey smell and taste of fresh-out-of-the-oven bread to millions of soldiers.

★ ★ ★

THAT "HOMEMADE" LOAF would soon all but disappear. Both world wars contributed to its demise. During the first, stubborn consumers were ordered to buy factory-made bread, because group preparation of food minimized use of fuel and other resources that could then be allocated to the war effort. In the second, food scarcity, vitamin enrichment, and low prices increased consumption of store-bought loaves by almost half. When the troops returned home in 1945 and 1946, rather than scale back now that their military buyers had disappeared, companies focused their marketing efforts on the consumer. Overburdened housewives— and what housewife isn't?—were happy to oblige.

America's appetite for bread—the whiter and fluffier, the better— was never heartier; in the 1950s, the food accounted for almost a third of people's daily calories. Many parts of its manufacture were now mechanized and new bulk dough-making methods adopted, but bread, with its need for individual batches and long periods of rest, as well as its aversion to being either pumped or pressurized, was a culinary throwback—the antithesis of the modern factory and its implacable pro- duction line. Tinkerers began tinkering, and in the mid-1950s a new equipment design appeared, the Wallace & Tiernan Do-Maker, which eliminated the whole pesky fermentation business altogether, along with the need for the human touch.

Instead of mixing individual bowls of dough, a pool of perma-yeast— a slurry of yeast, yeast food (mineral salts and enzymes that help break down complex sugars into simple ones), and water—was created and continuously squirted into the flour. This blend was then briefly but violently mixed—from three to five minutes—shaped into loaves, left for a short while, and then cooked. Total time for the microbes to do their magic: fifty minutes of final "proofing" right before the loaf was placed on a conveyor belt and carried into the oven. Compare that to the four to six hours of rising that occurred with earlier factory bread-making methods, and to the twelve to sixteen hours in traditional bakeries.*

A few things were lost in this new process—namely flavor, aroma, and texture—all of which were attributable to a long slow rise, according to none other than the army. "The normal ingredients of bread . . . are all mild in flavor, as is a freshly mixed dough. The tremendous complex of enzymatic reactions during fermentation gives rise to the formation of many new substances sufficiently volatile to produce olfactory stimuli. The actual baking process, in the course of which crust is formed at a temperature which may reach 150°C, while the loaf interior approaches the boiling temperature of water, engenders many new reaction products which contribute greatly to flavor."[4]

The textural issues in mechanically developed dough were even worse. First, the gluten molecules reacted poorly to the savage beating they received in "mixing," breaking some of the bonds between strands, which contributed to a cakier texture and lower height. To mimic the complex network of proteins formed during traditional rising-kneading-rising, bakers switched to higher-protein wheat varieties, added gluten during milling, and sometimes even during dough preparation. (In fact, there's a whole industry built on the production of "vital wheat gluten," which is also used in vegetarian meat substitutes, pet food, and, increasingly, as a binder, filler, or protein fortification in other food products.)

---

* In 1961 in England, a similarly speedy bread-making technique dependent on "mechanical dough development," the Chorleywood Bread Process, appeared. It is widely used in Britain and former British colonies, but because it uses low-protein wheat isn't suitable for the high-protein wheat grown in the United States and Canada (high protein is needed precisely to withstand the mechanical mauling it receives in manufacturing).

Second, the bread didn't rise enough. This was due in part to the drastically shortened proofing period, which didn't give naturally occurring enzymes as much time to break down the starch. It was also because of a historic shift in flour composition. In preindustrial farming, sheaves of wheat were left in the field to cure. Some of the grains began to germinate, which increases the presence of enzymes, in both the grain and the milled flour. To address these deficiencies, industrial bread makers added malted barley—malting is when you let seeds germinate before drying them—to increase the enzyme content of the flour.

Enzymes are monomaniacs, proteins on the prowl for a particular substance or substances; when they find it, they facilitate one specific chemical reaction—over and over and over again. This may not sound like much, but in fact they speed up regular organic chemistry by factors of millions, billions, or more. All living cells have enzymes, and organisms from different kingdoms can have the same (or a very similar) enzyme; for example, amylase, which breaks up starch molecules, is found in fungi, bacteria, plants, animals, and your mouth and pancreas. In traditional bread, there are two sources of amylase enzymes: the wheat and the yeast. Both snip up starch molecules into the short sugar chains that nourish the yeast that excretes the carbon dioxide that makes the bread rise.

Amylase was the first enzyme ever to be isolated, from malted barley in 1833. This was no accident; the protein was vitally important to three large industries: as a component of malted wheat or barley flour, it was the principal way breweries, distilleries, and bakeries broke down starch into sugar, feeding the yeast that made their products. In Japan, sake was brewed using the same enzyme—but from a mold, *Aspergillus oryzae*. Thought to have originated in China two to three thousand years ago, *koji*, as the fungus is called, was used and sold commercially in Japan from the thirteenth century or so on. In 1894 Jokichi Takamine, an immigrant taking inspiration from the libations of his native country, received the first U.S. biotech patent for the industrial production of fungal alpha-amylase. His hope was that American distillers would take to the more powerful starch digester. They didn't, but he did manage to license his process to Parke, Davis & Company, a Detroit pharmaceutical company, which merchandised it as a treatment for dyspepsia. (With these riches and those from a later venture involving adrenaline, Takamine purchased Washington, D.C.'s famous cherry trees.) Later improvements in enzyme production technology, in particular moving from time-and-space-consuming surface to submerged fermentation, and the increasingly widespread use of bacterial amylases (which tolerate neutral and alkaline pH) in textile and paper businesses to clean up residual starch, paved the way for a lateral hop to the bakery industry.

Army research into preserving bread began in earnest during World War II, when soldier complaints about hardtack and crackers that accompanied battle rations reached a crescendo, but the technical difficulties were so great that nothing was fielded. By the early 1950s, this endeavor was going full bore: of the forty grain and cereal research projects listed in the 1952–53 *Survey of Food and Nutrition Research in the United States of America,* eleven were related to the Quartermaster Corps' goal of producing shelf-stable bread. (Another nineteen were devoted to the army's other major area of interest, the development of baking mixes with dried flour, leavening, and other ingredients; these gave rise to commercial quick bread, muffin, and cake mixes.) A phalanx of researchers at the Quartermaster Food and Container Institute for the Armed Forces, other government laboratories, universities, and food companies around the country were enlisted to study bread flavor, browning, molding, and staling.

A novel idea to keep bread fresh was proposed by a small laboratory founded by the biochemist James S. Wallerstein, a frequent wartime Quartermaster Corps collaborator and the scion of a family that owned an early twentieth-century malt- and hops-processing business. "Widespread use of the recent important development of canned bread is limited to a large extent by the staling of the bread in the cans. Although such canned bread may remain fresh for some time, it firms up eventually and becomes stale in the can. I have found that bread, baked by my process in which the dough contains heat-stable amylolytic enzymes [bacterial amylases], can be canned and still not undergo this crumb staling or firming which heretofore has prevented the widespread use of this canning process."[5] In the early 1950s the Department of Grain Industry at Kansas State College (later University) was tapped to further experiment with how fungal and bacterial enzymes might be applied to baked goods to prolong freshness. (The Fleischmann Laboratories also did some work on bacterial amylases in baked goods and published a paper on the topic in 1953.) The Kansas State team included Max Milner, who had spent the war years at Pillsbury working on rations; John Johnson, a baking technologist; Byron Miller, a chemist and a World War II veteran; and several others. In 1955 Johnson published "Fungal Enzymes in Baking" in *Baker's Digest.* A couple of years later, Johnson and a colleague produced a special report on one of their Quartermaster Corps contracts, "Determination of the Feasibility of Producing Non-Staling Bread-like Products," in which they used both a fatty acid (these molecular chains occur naturally or can be synthesized; they are essential components of fats) and a bacterial amylase to produce a three-day-old bread with a "60% softer crumb," although they doubted that very long-term storage—two to four weeks—would be feasible. All alpha-amylases not only increase the sugar available for yeast fermentation but also help to soften crumb and increase volume. Fungal amylases, however, like their source organism, prefer it cool and are inactivated by cooking; bacterial alpha-amylase tolerates heat and a portion will continue to function after baking, keeping the bread texture soft for days or weeks. Fifty years later, Kansas State University boasts of this discovery as a "major research [contribution] . . . to the field of grain science and grain processing."

> In 1953, B.S. Miller, J.A. Johnson and D.L. Palmer published a journal article in which they showed that bacterial alpha-amylase was a potent inhibitor of crumb firming in bread, although their source of enzyme also caused the bread crumb to be sticky. That work confirmed a claim by S.S. Jackel and coworkers at the 1952 AACC [American Association of Cereal Chemists] National Meeting that bacterial amylase could be used to retard the staling

of bread. Today, so-called maltogenic alpha-amylase is used to inhibit bread firming for weeks, resulting in huge savings in the cost of delivering bread to the marketplace.[6]

As is always the case, before a scientific breakthrough can become a lucrative business, a number of technical issues needed to be resolved—in this instance, not new and better machines, but new and better laboratory processes. There were three important ones for industrial enzyme production. The first, which dates back to the late 1940s, was microfiltration, or ultrafiltration, membranes. As a project to copycat German technology, funded by the army at the California Institute of Technology, the filters were originally developed to test drinking water, but in the 1960s and 1970s their use was extended to biotech applications. The second was cell immobilization, the most common technique of which is implanting the cell in a sticky substrate, a process invented in the early 1960s. The final innovation was genetic engineering; the first successful recombinant DNA and transgenic organisms were created in the early 1970s. By the 1980s the stars had aligned, and the biotechnology industry took off—and with it industrial enzyme production for foods and beverages. In 1990 the first genetically modified enzyme—host organism: *Bacillus stearothermophilus* from an Icelandic hot spring—to prolong the freshness and increase the softness of bakery products without their becoming gummy was launched.

Today almost all supermarket breads are conditioned with microbial enzymes, especially bacterial ones, which soften texture, increase volume, add color, and extend shelf life by one or two weeks. This was a godsend for industrial bakers. Since the 1960s consumers have been increasingly suspicious of chemical additives and governments stricter in their regulation of ingredients. Because enzymes are a "processing aid" that leaves virtually no residue, they are considered "clean label," meaning they are not required to be listed on the block of print on the packaging. Besides all sorts of bakery items, enzymes are used to make sugar syrups, including the much-vilified high-fructose corn syrup, as well as to filter juices, clarify alcoholic beverages, speed ripening of and add flavor to cheese, create lactose-free milk, and tenderize meat. In the 1990s a market for these biotech ingredients emerged, dominated then and now by Swedish giant Novozymes. The global enzyme business currently earns more than $5 billion annually, of which roughly a third is for food and beverage additives.

All these changes may be a recipe for ill health. The modern loaf has more gluten to withstand mechanical dough development, more yeast to compensate for the lack of rising time, and a less developed fermentation than the loaves of the past. Exogenous enzymes make up the difference. Recent spikes in autoimmune disorders such as Crohn's and intestinal dysfunctions such as celiac disease (CD) appear linked to changes in bread. The authors of a global overview of Crohn's pose this question: "What unites Canterbury in New Zealand, Nova Scotia and Manitoba in Canada, Amiens in France, Maastricht in the Netherlands, Stockholm in Sweden, and Minnesota in the US . . . ?" Here, perhaps, is a clue: sufferers have antibodies for *Saccharomyces cerevisiae*, baker's yeast (although the microbes are inactivated by cooking). And here's another: they are some of the places where people eat the most industrial bread, according to Euromonitor International, a market research company.

Likewise, there has been a worldwide jump in CD. Because this is a reaction to wheat, it's not surprising that countries where wheat is a staple have high rates of the illness; what is surprising is its occurrence has increased over time. The authors of a 2013 worldwide review of the condition note that "an 'epidemic' of CD was described in Sweden from 1985 to 1995, possibly related to a doubling of gluten content in baby food at that time."[7] Some of the natural enzymes in yeast break down flour proteins—in particular gliadin, the component of gluten associated with CD. But with their abbreviated rising times and added wheat protein, finished loaves undoubtedly now have more gluten—and thus gliadin—than ever before. Could the increase in prevalence of CD be related to the higher gluten contents of industrial breads?

We eat it for breakfast, we eat it for lunch, very occasionally we eat it right out of the bag, but does this stuff—immature dough whipped up with air and inoculated with exogenous enzymes—really deserve the name bread at all, one of the holy trinity of fermented foods, along with beer/wine and cheese? To step into that particular breach, we have the French, with their indefatigable knack for proclamations, whose 1993 *Décret Pain,* among other edicts (no freezing, no additives), orders that real bread be composed of a dough "fermented using baker's yeast [*S. cerevisiae*]." By this standard, all those neatly packaged loaves in the supermarket—the farmhouse white, the 100 percent whole wheat, the multigrain—which have risen only fifty minutes, are not bread. What are they? In the words of the army-funded contractors whose 1950s research on enzymes helped to create them, they are "non-staling bread-like products."

★ ★ ★

THERE'S A REASON WHY BAKERS ARE BLEARY-EYED; their wares need to be replenished daily. The traditional loaf has a lopsided relationship with time. On the front end, the dough lolls about for hours or even a day. On the back end, it must be eaten quickly or ends up stale. For manufacturers, the trick to profitability is to shorten the first period and extend the second (not for your benefit but theirs—to reduce unsalable product). For the military, this became a necessity in 1991, the year the army switched from canned to plastic-pouch-encased rations.

Although it was not well liked, beginning in the Korean War and continuing through Vietnam, the Quartermaster Corps had finally produced a tinned bread to accompany the combat ration. The trick had been the rigid, metal cylinder, which acted like a minioven, allowing the dough to expand during processing, and kept it from being crushed afterward. The new multilayer plastic and foil pouches offered no such protection, transmitting the pressure of water and crushing the delicate carbon dioxide–riddled gluten network—bread is, technically, a foam— into a dense, inedible mass. Cooking in the cans also eliminated bacterial contamination, because they were sealed before cooling enough to support a beachhead invasion from new microorganisms. Suddenly, everything the army had laboriously developed in the years during and after World War II to create a palatable slice or two had to be unceremoniously scrapped.

Foreseeing this day, Natick had been working since the mid-1980s on an extended-shelf-life pouch bread, among other things, using a new technique called hurdle technology, which had been developed for the German army for food that hasn't been heat-sterilized. The approach combines multiple mild barriers to microbial growth, such as water activity, acidity, and chemical reactivity, with chilling, heat sterilization, and other factors. While the bread Natick developed wasn't going to fell recruits with botulism, it still did what old bread always did: the crust got soft, the crumb got hard, and that delicious olfactory advertisement, its yeasty, caramelized aroma, dissipated.

Understanding the physical and chemical changes bread undergoes as it ages is a problem that has bedeviled scientists for well over a century. From a 1940 article in *Cereal Chemistry:* "Present knowledge as to the nature of the staling process is inadequate, and further strictly controlled scientific researches are necessary to determine the nature of this process before looking for substances that will prevent it." From a 1981 review in *Cereal Chemistry:* "The consensus among the various workers and studies still appears to be that changes in starch play the major role in bread firmness. Bread staling, however, is an extremely complex phenomenon and is difficult to define in straightforward terms." From a 2003 overview in *Comprehensive Reviews in Food Science and Food Safety:* "The molecular basis of staling is examined. . . . The conclusion reached is that bread staling is a complex phenomenon in which multiple mechanisms operate. . . . The key hindrance to development of a preventive strategy for bread staling is the failure to understand the mechanism of the process."

Amazingly little is known for sure. Many factors contribute to the staling of bread, including the redistribution of water between the gluten matrix and the starch. But most agree that it has to do primarily with changes to the two starch molecules, amylopectin (70–80 percent of wheat starch) and amylose (20–30 percent). In the uncooked starch granule, the two kinds of molecules form helices, with the amylopectin packed together in repeating patterns, while the amylose remains disorganized. During baking, these granules become swollen with water, the helix loosens, and some amylose leaches out. Immediately after baking, however, the amylose hijacks some of the nearby water molecules and crystallizes in a process called retrogradation. This process redistributes the moisture in the bread and is believed to be largely complete by the time it has cooled to room temperature. The amylopectin crystallizes much more slowly, over a period of days, but perhaps because it is present in a greater proportion, its retrogradation is more noticeable, making the bread seem dry, although in fact it may have the same total moisture content as before. But that's about where scientific agreement on staling ends.

This uncertainty has given rise to the let's-just-throw-stuff-at-it school of bread-shelf-life science. Emulsifiers, which affect the cooking and swelling properties of starch? Go for it. Surfactants, which retard water penetration and swelling? Sure, why not? Gums and hydrocolloids, which add stability, softness, and mouthfeel? Can't hurt. And then, of course, there are the bacterial amylases—who knows exactly why they work, but they do, so in they go. This was the approach taken by the Natick Center in trying to tackle the issue of staling in its new pouch bread. The team, consisting of Daniel Berkowitz and Lauren Oleksyk, then a recent graduate of the Framingham State food-science program, began work on the problem in the mid-1980s. "That's what I did every day with Dan for a couple years," says Oleksyk. "Every day I'd come in; we'd meet and look at the formulas we'd done the day before. We'd see what worked and what didn't. Every day, we were tweaking ingredients, making up new prototypes, storing them. We always looked at texture, color, aroma, taste."

Eventually, they hit on a technique—combining an emulsifier and a hydrocolloid, a thickening gum made of long chains of molecules that evenly disperse in liquid—that seemed to work miracles. "What we added was not done anywhere else," explains Oleksyk. "We knew that sucrose ester was an emulsifier in a lot of products. Well, we combined that with PVP, an ingredient which although it has GRAS [generally recognized as safe] status, isn't usually used in commercial baking. [Polyvinylpyrrolidone is a synthetic polymer that passes through the body without being digested; its typical use is as a binder and coating for pills.] We didn't know it would have the effect it would have. . . . We found things that we just didn't expect: the softness, the volume. We knew it had a water-binding effect. But we weren't expecting it to affect nonenzymatic browning as much as it did. And whiteness. I changed the percentages so many times, I filled an entire notebook with the different formulations, probably 150 or more. Since then, we took PVP out and used other things to get the shelf life, but that was the original patent."

In the particulars, the Natick approach to preventing bread staling was hit or miss, but it was roughly based on a new theory about how to understand food—one borrowed from polymer science. This did not, as had been done in the past, view food solely as innumerable individual chemical reactions, crucially affected by temperature, time, water, and oxygen, but also as a unified system with its own characteristics and reactions. As individual molecules have phase transitions, the temperatures when solids change to liquids and liquids to gas, collections of disorganized but interacting molecules—called amorphous solids in chemistry terminology—have glass transitions, the temperatures at which they change from brittle to rubbery to liquid. Glass is one such system (hence the name); its components are molten at about 2,400°F; if cooled a couple of thousand degrees rather quickly, they become increasingly viscous, but the molecules never lock into place. Food and food components are others. This similarity was first noticed by candy engineers in the mid-1960s, but the concept wasn't applied to other edibles with any regularity until the 1980s.

Although various university scientists worked on the idea, the most prolific—and vociferous—advocates were a duo at Nabisco, Louise Slade and Harry Levine. Their early careers had been at General Foods, a century-old conglomerate—General Foods was merged with Kraft in 1989 and their food businesses combined in 1995—where Slade had worked on frozen dough, and Levine on frozen desserts. Both of these foods exhibit the same changes as polymers as the temperature drops, becoming more viscous, then hardening and eventually "collapsing." (In the other kind of solids, crystalline solids, molecules are locked into regular repeating patterns; because they're already in their lowest energy state, they're not affected much by chilling.) In an amorphous solid, lower temperatures reduce the energy available to hold the disparate and disorganized molecules together; eventually these bonds break to find less demanding arrangements. Perhaps it was this observation that led the pair to polymer science and one of their first published papers together, "A Food Polymer Science Approach to the Practice of Cryostabilization Technology." They've since racked up several hundred and are the leading authorities in the field.

In Slade and Levine's model, as stored food experienced time- and temperature-related physical and chemical deterioration, its glass transition temperature could change. This means that if the food item had been crisp, its glass transition temperature might drop from above to below room temperature, and it could become limp or soggy. If it had been moist, its glass transition temperature might fall still more, allowing increased mobility of its components, resulting in crystallizations. If we apply this idea to aging bread, the retrograding starch molecules capture some of the water, so less is available overall, raising the glass transition temperature and creating a hard, stale crumb. Slade and Levine also determined the glass transition temperatures of the system in the presence of a range of additives, which could then be used as needed, depending on the desired characteristics of the food. It was this idea that Berkowitz and Oleksyk put to work in their formulation for shelf-stable bread.

However, it was still more of a concept than an application, which left too much guesswork in the lab. The Natick Center asked Pavinee Chinachoti, a University of Massachusetts food chemist, to do studies that might explain the underlying staling mechanism, would allow them to measure starch gelatinization and retrogradation, and predict the effect on shelf life of different combinations of ingredients. Chinachoti worked with Natick for more than a decade, eventually editing one of the two textbooks on the topic, *Bread Staling*. As part of this work,

Chinachoti and her Natick counterpart, Linnea Hallberg, often described the remarkable results Natick had had with their nonstaling MRE bread, as well as a whole family of related products, including the shelf-stable sandwich.

Smelling potential profits, Nabisco asked for a piece of the prize. In 1996 the company invited Natick to enter into a Cooperative Research and Development Agreement (CRADA). The blue-chip conglomerate, whose existing business was mostly crackers and cookies, with a couple of intermediate-moisture items such as granola bars, would get to go up close and personal with Natick's invention; Natick might get some pointers on how to make its extended-life bakery items tastier, or perhaps even gain a manufacturer of the product. The group was a large one on both sides, and from Nabisco included both Slade and Levine, as well as a microbiologist, Martin Cole, now chief of the Australian national science agency's Division of Animal, Food and Health Sciences. Says Cole, "At the heart of [the shelf-stable sandwich] was an understanding of the starch retrogradation. . . . Part of the CRADA was to understand the mechanism behind the Natick work, and then come up with other commercially more viable methods to prevent crystallization of starch." Which was a polite way of saying that the army's choice of antistaling additives—PVP and sucrose esters, later xanthan and guar gum, and still later 6 percent glycerol solution, according to Slade—might alienate customers. The Nabisco scientists came up with an alternative set of additives and went into the pilot kitchen.

It may have needed some adjusting, but the idea of the shelf-stable bread, especially with a filling, was a "platform"—food company speak for a basic recipe from which dozens of variations could be created— with legs. "The approach and the data that they had were very useful in terms of designing new products," explains Cole. "Essentially what it did was allowed us to knock out an operating space and saved us a lot of work to understand where the edges of this thing were. Based on that we were able to put some products across a framework, different combinations of things, different moistures. . . . The work that Natick had done gave two things. It gave us insight into the mechanistic aspect of staling. Also, it helped position the right elements and other combinations of things that might prevent staling." Nabisco's prototypes included a whole range of savory and sweet bakery items that tasted "pretty good" and could remain on shelves for months at a time.

They never made it to the market. In 2000, as part of the continuing tobacco industry liability shell game, Nabisco sold all its food brands to tobacco giant Philip Morris, which merged them with those of Kraft (now Mondelēz) and General Foods, which it had acquired earlier. Then Nabisco, which had previously merged with and then spun out R.J. Reynolds and that now had no real business, sold itself, along with all its cigarette-related liability, to R.J. Reynolds. Lost in the shuffle, along with the corporate responsibility to pay any new personal injury claims, was Nabisco's research on extended-shelf-life bread products. Kraft, as new corporate overlords are wont to do, put in place its own research goals and repopulated the Nabisco labs with its own staff. But good ideas, once let loose, don't die, they just keep knocking on doors until someone lets them in. Today, treating food as a polymer and manipulating its glass transition temperature by the judicious selection of additives is an accepted part of product design, and used in everything from encapsulated ingredients, frozen foods, baby foods, pasta, energy bars, snack foods, bakery items, candy, powders, to extruded cereal products (that pretty much describes 75 percent of the American diet right there), and even to breakfast cereals with add-ins.

CHEESE PURISTS THE WORLD over exalt their mummified milk. Their silken Goudas and savory Emmentalers. Their fetid fetas and squeaky queso frescos. Their moldy Roqueforts and runny Camemberts. These disks of rotted dairy are the pinnacle of thousands of years of experimentation that began when a herdsman carrying a ruminant's stomach brimming with milk found that by journey's end, he had a bag full of curds and whey.

Modern cheese making is a little more complicated, but the same principles apply. Fresh milk is allowed to ferment, with either wild or cultured bacteria, typically one of the friendly LABs (lactic acid bacteria). Then, when they have raised the acidity enough, rennet—enzymes from calves' stomachs (these have now been replaced with laboratory-produced enzymes)—is added. This coagulates the caseins, which make up about 80 percent of the total milk protein, so that they form a gel. Then there's a lot of manipulation—cutting, stirring, and heating—that removes fluid, or whey, leaving behind solid curds. The curds are put into molds, salted or brined, and pressed, which expels more whey and turns the cheese into a solid mass. Mold may be added, either at the beginning or later in the process. Then, depending on the variety, the cheeses are matured for anywhere from two weeks to two years, allowing enzymes, both those from microbes and those from the rennet, to turn fats and proteins into tasty new substances.

Cheese is one of the bedrocks on which the Western diet is founded—a long-term storage method for excess milk, especially when cool storerooms and caves were available. But the food didn't fare so well during summer or in hot climates. With heat, animal fat softens or even liquefies, oozing out and creating an oily and unappealing mess. In the early twentieth century, dairymen on either side of the Atlantic—the Swiss pair Walter Gerber and Fritz Stettler in 1911 and James Kraft in 1916—hit on and patented a solution to the seasonal sweats: emulsifying salts. The chemical disperses water-phobic caseins by exchanging sodium for calcium; this permits the now smaller particles to be diffused and suspended in liquid. Melting traditional cheeses and mixing them with the emulsifying salts resulted in a cheese-like product that withstands high temperatures and protracted storage. Even better, this new food could be made and sold very cheaply, because it could be produced, at least in part, from the rinds and irregular bits left over from cutting wheels of cheese into bricks. Melting the ingredients also pasteurized them, inactivating the live bacteria and enzymes and contributing to a longer shelf life.

The army placed its first order for processed cheese—which at the beginning, came in only one flavor: white—during World War I, buying twenty-five million quarter-pound tins from Kraft. This single act probably established Kraft's century-long (and still going strong) food industry hegemony. By the time World War II rolled around, the military was a raving cheeseaholic, consuming the dairy product by itself, on sandwiches, or as sauces for vegetables, potatoes, and pasta. In 1944 alone, the Quartermaster Corps bought more than one hundred million pounds from Kraft's parent company, National Dairy Products Corporation (which finally itself took the Kraft name in 1969), as well as five hundred thousand pounds of cheese spread (bacon bits optional) to accompany the K and some of the C rations. During the war, the company's sales almost doubled. But it still wasn't enough. The military was hungry for new ways to store, ship, and eat cheese.

At the beginning of the war, the army had embarked on a dehydration-and-compression spree—by removing heavy water and reducing its volume, more food could be packed into a single shipment, always an advantage when there are millions of mouths to feed. All foodstuffs except meat were run through the drying chambers and squashed into bricks—fruits and vegetables, flour, potatoes, eggs, and cheese. As would become its historic pattern, the military funded or supported a variety of efforts, some of which were destined to die a quiet death and others that would garner glory, becoming wartime staples and the basis for future consumer products. Cheese dehydration research was conducted by the Quartermaster Corps' Subsistence Research Laboratory, through the USDA laboratories, at various universities, including the University of California at Davis, and by industry, notably Kraft. Unless a food has a strong and flexible internal structure—think cellulose, the long chains of sugar molecules that give plant cells their rigidity—it crumbles when it dries out, something food technologists call *fines.* One can imagine the first experiment in drying and pressing a proud block of Wisconsin cheddar: cheese dust. This ruled out eating reconstituted cheese out of hand in slices or chunks. But for cooking, the granular form would be an advantage.

The first real cheese powder was developed in 1943 by George Sanders, a USDA dairy scientist. (Even before the war began, USDA's research facilities had been enlisted to work toward military goals, exhorted by

Secretary of Agriculture Henry Wallace "to consider their possible contributions to national needs as the defense program approaches the stage of 'maximum effort.'"[8] This relationship continues to this day; the USDA has collaborated with the Quartermaster Corps and later the Natick Center on topics as varied as chemical testing, fungi collection and classification, potatoes, dairy, and, from 1980 on, operation of the army's radiation food sterilization program.) Until then, it had been "considered impossible to dehydrate natural, fat-containing cheese,"[9] because the heat melted the fat, which then separated out. Sanders's innovation was to divide the process into two steps. In the first, the cheese, shredded or grated, was dried at a low temperature; this hardened the surface proteins of the particles, forming a protective barrier around the lipids. Once sufficient water had been evaporated, the cheese was ground and dehydrated at a higher temperature. The final step was to form it into what the patent describes as cakes. A 1943 war bond ad unveiled the product to the public with a picture of a bare-chested soldier feeding a second soldier bundled up in a parka with a cheese cake on a pointy stick:

> For jungle or ski troops—a new kind of cheese! . . . But they should taste the same—and taste *good*—wherever they're eaten. That has meant many headaches for the Army Quartermaster Corps and the food processors who supply them. . . . For emergency use in arctic and tropics, National Dairy laboratories developed a dehydrated, compressed cheese that keeps well anywhere and takes less shipping weight and space.

In the summer of 1945, Little Boy and Fat Man were detonated in Japan, ending the war and leaving the Quartermaster Corps with warehouses full of food as well as an elaborate manufacturing and distribution system still churning out goods for millions of troops. This would take years to redirect or dismantle. Fearful of the effect of the sudden withdrawal of its huge wartime contracts, the government propped up the dairy business first by buying its excess product and then, in some cases, by selling it back to the same producers at lower prices. (The

Commodity Credit Corporation, created during the Great Depression and still in existence, would later distribute these surpluses to welfare recipients and the elderly—the storied "government cheese.") A temporary federal agency, the Surplus Property Administration, sold off at bargain-basement prices the food the Quartermaster Corps had amassed.

Who doesn't love something they get for free or at a third of the original cost?[10] But what could one do with football fields full of potato flakes, a cave stuffed with dried eggs (the army's strange storage location for one hundred million pounds of the stuff), or a mountain of dehydrated cheese? Well, there was one group always interested in lowering the cost of finicky fresh ingredients: the grocery manufacturers, businesses such as Swift, Quaker Oats, General Foods, General Mills, Libby's, Borden, McCormick, Colgate-Palmolive, Gerber, Scott Paper, Kellogg's, Pillsbury, and Kraft. (The strength of the companies that produced the packaged goods that lined the nation's nascent supermarkets, many with deep military ties, only grew over the next century, as did that of their trade group, the Grocery Manufacturers Association, today the food industry's most powerful lobbying organization.) Perhaps instead of real cheese, the food corporations could mix in the cheap powder to add flavor. Not only would they save outright on the cost of ingredients, they'd pay a lot less to ship and store them—after all, that was the army's primary purpose in developing dehydrated cheese in the first place. These ration conversions inspired a flood of fledgling products, particularly in the new and growing categories of convenience and snack foods.

In 1948 the Frito Company (it merged with H. W. Lay & Company in 1961 to become Frito-Lay, Inc.) debuted the country's first cheesy snack food, made with the same Wisconsin cheddar the army used for its dehydrated products. Frito Company founder Charles Doolin had been a military supplier, even building a facility in San Diego, where there is a naval base, to service his contracts. According to his daughter Kaleta Doolin, "During the war, tins of chips were sent overseas to be served in mess halls and sold in PXs. This venture helped put the company over the top as a nationwide business."[11] Afterward, new plants were opened in Dallas, Los Angeles, and Salt Lake City, where soon cornmeal and water were being extruded, puffed, fried in oil, and coated with finger-licking, orange dehydrated cheese. Cheetos! Other companies quickly followed suit, producing savory curls, doodles, and puffs.

Today, the cheese powder category has expanded to include a variety of natural cheeses; extended cheese with additional ingredients such as stabilizers, milk solids, and emulsifying salts; and concentrated enzyme-modified cheese, which is used primarily as a flavoring agent. Dehydrated cheese permeates our lives, enlivening everything from beloved basics such as boxed mac 'n' cheese to the school of Goldfish that swim through our childhoods and the addictive white or orange dust with which Frito-Lay and other food producers continue to coat their many snack foods. The military's World War II invention, intended to help nourish warriors in battle, became one of the seminal snack and industrial food ingredients of the twentieth century and is still going strong in the new millennium.

Chapter 10

PLASTIC PACKAGING REMODELS THE PLANET

LUNCH BOX ITEMS #6 AND #7: SARAN WRAP AND JUICE POUCHES

"Girls! It's 9:30 p.m.! Time for bed." I save my Word document, shut the window with the—blush—*Daily Mail,* and put the stack of bills next to my laptop as a reminder to pay them tomorrow. (Computer, olefin carpet, cables, phone.) The front door creaks open. "Smokey! Kitty!" Eloisa, our youngest, stays up worrying unless the cat's in. She runs upstairs to join her sister Dalila in the bathroom, where they stand together at the sink, brushing their teeth. (Toothbrushes; all those three-quarter-empty shampoos, lotions, and sprays; latex house paint; PVC plumbing.) I climb the three flights of stairs from my basement office to their room in the attic. Tucked under hibiscus-print quilts, they are both reading. Smokey lies across the foot of Eloisa's bed, purring. Across the hall, my mother sits in an armchair, also reading. In the kitchen, we hear clinking and clattering. It's trash night, and my husband is wrestling closed two large garbage bags, regular and recycling, filled mostly with the detritus from the river of plastic that runs silently through our house. (Plastic bags, metallicized bags, plastic films, laminated foil-and-plastic pouches, plastic-coated cardboard, plastic clamshells, plastic tubs, plastic bottles.) I plant a kiss on one soft cheek. "Good night, sweetie." And then the other. "Good night, sweetie." Later, I'll text our college-age daughter the same thing. As I head downstairs, Jorge comes in, the tumbler clicking into place as he locks the door behind him. Another day ended, and we're all safe. Benediction.

★ ★ ★

IF YOU'D TOLD AN EGYPTIAN MORTICIAN or a Babylonian boat maker that the twentieth and twenty-first centuries would be built of pitch, he would have guffawed heartily. Ancient civilizations collected sticky black bitumen, or asphalt, which welled up spontaneously in rocky Middle Eastern outcrops, and put it to use as paving for roads, mortar for building, glue, weatherproofing, and an embalming agent. But beyond that, the sludge wasn't good for much. In fact, no one paid petroleum much mind until 1879, when a German engineer, Karl Benz, successfully harnessed a combustion engine to a carriage. Suddenly consumption of crude oil, the refining of which had been invented in 1848 by the Scottish chemist James Young, who noticed that heat caused oil to seep from the roof of a coal mine, skyrocketed—and kept climbing, in the United States increasing more than two hundred times during the twentieth century.[1] Still, after the precious fuel had been distilled, there was the issue of sludge. Then oil company engineers, in an effort to beat the competition with better-running gasoline, began to further refine crude petroleum by separating the spontaneous-combustion-prone heavier hydrocarbons. These waste products eventually became the signature material of the modern age: plastic.

There are some people who always seem to land on their feet. The Austrian chemist Herman Mark, the father of polymer—colloquially, plastics—science, was one of them. This is not so much luck as skill—one that combines unceasing work at one's profession, the careful cultivation of connections, and the ability to make life-changing decisions in an instant. Mark had all this and more: he was athletic, courageous, and optimistic, a formidable man who would be tested and triumph not once but several times during his life.

Just out of his teens, he managed to become a decorated soldier and earn a doctorate—rising early even if he'd drunk his companions under the table the night before. Wounded by shrapnel in the ankle as a young Austrian army soldier in World War I, he read chemistry textbooks as he recovered. Later in the conflict, he was captured, but after six months bribed his way to freedom to visit his sick father. Once at home in Austria, Mark matriculated at the University of Vienna, breezing through his much-postponed Ph.D. in chemistry in less than two years. He was promptly invited by Fritz Haber—whose discovery of how to synthesize ammonia revolutionized both agriculture (fertilizer) and warfare (explosives) and whose development of the deadly chlorine gas used in the war gained him the epithet "the Father of Chemical Weapons"—to work at the newly formed Kaiser Wilhelm Institute for Textile Fiber Research in Berlin. There, the young scientist quickly mastered X-ray crystallography, a technique then in its infancy in which the structures of atoms and molecules are mapped by bouncing high-energy electromagnetic waves off them.

Mark's newfound laboratory skills allowed him to settle one of the most heated controversies in his field. Chemists had made huge advances during the nineteenth and early twentieth centuries: identifying the elements, decoding atomic structure, and developing models for how molecules bonded. But the next step, understanding how these building blocks were assembled in more complex arrangements, had been hobbled by one man, Nobel Prize winner Emil Fischer, who'd dismissed out of hand the possibility of very large molecules. This eventually led to an intellectual showdown at the 1926 annual meeting of the Society for Natural Science and Medicine in Düsseldorf, Germany. First up were the organic chemists Hans Pringsheim and Max Bergmann, who argued that the phenomena were, in fact, colloids—clumps of floating but unbound particles. Then came Hermann Staudinger, the original proponent of the concept, who demonstrated new data on rubber and synthetic polymers and insisted that they, protein, and cellulose were all macromolecules. The audience remained unconvinced. The decisive moment came during Mark's presentation in which he shared his X-ray diffraction studies of cellulose, the compound that lends rigidity to plants, comparing it with the recently discovered structure of graphite and diamond, a large network held together by covalent bonds. At the end he affirmed that cellulose could, in fact, be a macromolecule. "Terrifying," said Richard Willstätter, chair of the debate. "But, on the basis of what we have heard today, it seems that I shall have to slowly adjust to this thought."[2] Shortly thereafter, Mark left the Kaiser Wilhelm Institute and accepted a dual position at a Frankfurt university and the I. G. Farben company, a German chemical conglomerate, where, as the head of a laboratory on fiber and film, he was charged with developing synthetic textiles, as well as working on the first synthetic rubber and polyvinyl chloride.

Synthetic polymers replicated in the lab—and later the factory—what chemists were observing about natural polymers: that they were immense chains of repeating units linked by a backbone of carbon atoms. In nature, macromolecules come from living creatures. In the lab, they do, too—except the creatures lived sixty million years ago. Most man-made polymers are created from hydrocarbons, the one-thousandth of dead plant and animal matter that, instead of entering the food chain, escapes or is born into the ocean. There, this organic debris is pushed slowly, very slowly, deep into the earth, where high temperatures energize the molecules and high pressure forces them closer together. The resulting new substances are hydrocarbon monomers—the building blocks of synthetic polymers.

Aside from fuel, these monomers are actually one of the important by-products of the modern oil refinery, an eerie maze of hissing and thumping tanks, tubes, valves, and engines, often occupying hundreds of acres or more. The machinery may look complicated, but the principles it employs aren't. By heating crude oil—and, as was discovered later, applying pressure and chemical catalysts—engineers take advantage of the different boiling points of the component hydrocarbons, separating them in various chambers. The remaining heavy molecules are then "cracked" into small ones for reprocessing. There are literally thousands of different types of hydrocarbons, each with its own distinct molecular weight and configuration and, thus, distinct properties. Synthetic polymers, or plastics as most people call them, are made by taking a lot of these identical monomers and then linking them all together with heat and/or chemical catalysts.

Mark's work at I. G. Farben came to an abrupt halt in 1932, when, nervous about the increasing influence of the Nazi Party, the plant's managing director suggested to the half-Jewish Mark that it might behoove him to look for a new job. Obligingly he decamped back to Austria, transplanting his research projects to the University of Vienna, where he set up the first polymer science curriculum. But Mark's return to his homeland was short-lived. In early 1938 he was arrested by the Nazis, and only got away with a bold plan: he purchased his passport, which had been confiscated by the police, with a year's salary, turned the rest of his life savings into platinum clothes hangers, and loaded the family in the car for a Swiss "ski vacation." He then wrote to a Canadian paper manufacturer that had expressed interested in employing him in its cellulose research lab. The family spent two years in a mill town sixty miles west of Montreal, until Mark, again taking advantage of a business contact, arranged for an opportunity to start anew through a consulting job with DuPont and an academic position at the Polytechnic Institute of Brooklyn.

The appointment would usher in the Plastic Age.

Until the late 1930s, the material world was a dangerous place. Most durable objects were heavy and sharp, made of wood, glass, ceramics, and metal, while the few disposable ones were made of paper, wax, and cloth. World War II changed all that. The enormous demands the military had for materials—for everything from shoe eyelets to tires to tents—and for which, in some cases, such as with natural rubber, supply was interrupted by the Japanese, spurred a frantic scientific race for substitutes. One of these was the synthetic rubber program, the second largest after the Manhattan Project, and until the announcement of the atomic bomb, considered to be "the greatest technical achievement of all time."[3] The research was conducted by, among others, the United States Rubber Company, the University of Chicago, the University of Minnesota, the University of Illinois, Cornell, Princeton, and the Polytechnic

Institute of Brooklyn. But although Herman Mark had worked on the two fake rubbers, Buna-N and Buna-S, when they were invented in Germany in the 1930s, he was only peripherally involved in the project.

Mark had more interesting fish to fry: developing artificial materials to replace the traditional ones used in the prosaic items of daily life, an endeavor that would earn him the nickname the "Father of Polymer Science" and spark the transformation of the Polytechnic Institute of Brooklyn into the premier polymer research organization in the nation (at the time, the only one). "When I looked from Canada on the United States," said Mark, "the question was whether there was any work on polymers going on in academia. The answer was: scattered, not organized. Speed [a researcher at the University of Chicago] worked on the synthesis of new monomers and new polymers. . . . There was North Carolina; work was done there on fiber strength, fiber elasticity. . . . National Bureau of Standards was working with rubber, but not with fibers; no synthesis, not the whole thing. . . . Our idea was that we were going to have an organized program here."[4]

His ambitions dovetailed perfectly with those of the government. According to a postwar National Institute of Standards and Technology report, "By 1941 sufficient knowledge was available to set up emergency specifications utilizing plastics in place of scarce metals in many Government purchases. With Navy and NACA [NASA's predecessor agency, the National Advisory Committee for Aeronautics] funds, research began on the properties and fabrication of these strong lightweight materials. . . . Among new plastic products sent for testing were helmet liners, resinous coatings used for protection of steel hardware, bayonet handles, Bureau-designed binocular housings, bugles, canteens, clock housings, compass dials, raincoats, food packaging, goggles, insect screening, shaving brushes, and aircraft housings."

Mark's first Polytechnic post was at the Shellac Research Bureau, something of a backwater. That switched once Pearl Harbor was attacked and the war officially began; Indian and Thai imports of the insect resin, often used to insulate electrical fixtures, were halted by the Japanese. Finding a synthetic version became urgent. "We got a tremendous lift immediately," explained Mark, "because we were working on products and problems which became extremely important for the conduct of the war. . . . Permeability and impermeability of films; synthesis and characterization of synthetic rubber; and Cordura [a synthetic fabric developed by DuPont]. With these three things we had very large programs from the Army and from the government; several million dollars."[5]

Mark quickly became part of the university's inner circle, one of three wartime research magnets—the others were specialists in aviation and electronics—who together increased Polytechnic Institute of Brooklyn's sponsored research program almost tenfold between the years 1942 and 1945. Those contracts, many of them restricted, were with the Office of Scientific Research and Development (OSRD), NACA, the Navy Research Bureau, and the Quartermaster Corps. (In 1944, the funding the Polytechnic Institute of Brooklyn received from the Quartermaster Corps was more than that for any other contractor, including such illustrious names as the University of Chicago, Columbia University, General Electric, Arthur D. Little, MIT, the Mellon Institute, and Monsanto.)[6] Each of these military agencies had a pressing need for Mark's—and his fast-growing stable of polymer experts'—scientific knowledge and technical know-how to create or perfect new fibers, films, and rubber for the war. But "the main project that Mark was running . . . was working on polymers that were of use in films and coatings," said Bruno Zimm, one of the chemists who worked for him.[7]

A polymer can be millions of times as big as water, carbon dioxide, and other common molecules. The importance of its size can be understood by imagining shaking a cardboard box full of marbles and one full of beach balls. Which move around more? Marbles. Polymers, because they are so big and bristling with shorter side chains, don't shift position as readily as smaller molecules, and tend to jam up, reducing flow. This accounts for their three most important properties: viscosity, elasticity, and strength.

These characteristics are affected by heat; how and how much depends on the type of polymer. For example, thermoset plastics can be locked into permanent position by cooking, which causes irreversible cross-linking of their side chains. Thermoplastics, on the other hand, can be softened and remolded many times; their side chains slide by one another without catching much. Polymers can be used singly or in combination to increase strength and flexibility of the end material. Plasticizers, other much smaller petroleum-based molecules, are commonly added as well. Think of them as the marbles in the example above. If you mixed the marbles with the beach balls, they would push the beach balls farther apart, so the oversize inflatables move around more easily. Plasticizers lower the glass transition temperature, the point at which all flow stops, so most polymers are flexible at room temperature or below. With films, which are thermoplastic, the resulting resins are then treated in different ways—blown, rolled, stretched, and coextruded (combined with other polymers in layers)—to achieve the desired hardness, flexibility, vapor and other gas resistance, longevity, opacity, and strength.

One of the polymers worked on by Mark and his team was an oily green substance that had been discovered almost a decade earlier in a Dow Chemical lab, when a technician found the residue at the bottom of a beaker where he'd been making a dry-cleaning chemical from chlorine. "It was very difficult to dissolve," said the accidental inventor, Ralph Wiley, who almost immediately took out a patent. "There was no chemical that would touch it."[8] Saran, a copolymer—two monomers blended together into a single structure—of vinylidene chloride and vinyl chloride, is both tough and extremely resistant to water and oxygen. Its commercial debut was as a fiber for lawn chairs and train seat covers in the late 1930s, but a year or two later, another technician, Wilbur Stephenson, developed a method for creating a vinylidene film.

The army immediately saw Saran's potential as a protective barrier, spraying it on engines, guns, and metal parts to prevent corrosion from water and salt during shipment overseas on open decks. Later in the war, when it became apparent that the various combinations of cellophane (a shiny, stiff film from plant fiber), waxed paper, and foil were inadequate for shielding rations from moisture, the Quartermaster Corps began to explore the possibility of making a food-contact film from Saran. To do so, however, it would have to find a way to make this auspicious material flexible and keep it from becoming brittle and opaque as it aged.

The project was carried out at both the Polytechnic Institute of Brooklyn and the Dow Chemical Company, which to this day dominates the market for the monomers for both vinylidene chloride and vinyl chloride. At the chemical company, the project was led by Raymond Boyer of the Physics Laboratory. "The other job that took most of my time dealt with the light and heat stability of Saran—which we called at that time 'Ventyloid,'" explained Louis C. Rubens, a chemist in the lab. "Ralph Wiley had been working on Saran. Light and heat stability were already identified as the key problems of that material. Two colleagues tackled that problem. Lorne A. Matheson and Ray Boyer. They knew it was photo-degradation. . . . But they really didn't know how to prevent it. . . . Photodecomposition was a key problem then, as far as Saran was concerned. . . . It was primarily an Edisonian research program that was initiated by Boyer and Matheson."[9]

Into that Edisonian fumble in the dark, Herman Mark inserted some scientific scaffolding. As Dr. R. H. Boundy, the company's vice president for research and development, described it, "he [put] a theoretical base under the things we in industry were doing by trial and error."[10] Among the restricted projects conducted at Brooklyn were various studies on vinyl polymers and copolymers, the family of plastics to which Saran belongs. A goal of this research was "to act as a stimulus by supplying new fundamental ideas which may eventually be utilized in a practical way by industrial laboratories. . . . The Laboratories have done much work with the overall aging characteristics of plastic films including such problems as plasticizer migration, sunlight and atmosphere degradation and freedom from blocking."[11]

In 1946 the Chemistry Department of the University of Buffalo held a symposium to disseminate the work on vinyl polymers and plasticizers during the war and invited chemists from both Polytechnic and Dow. In his opening address, E. F. Izard of DuPont lauded the government's effort to come up with new materials for flexible sheeting and films to replace rubber and cellophane, which were either unavailable for or inadequate to wartime tasks.

> The critical military requirements soon made it evident that only polyvinyl butyral, polyvinyl chloride, and copolymers of vinyl chloride with other vinyl compounds [such as Saran], would be suitable substitutes [for flexible sheeting]. . . . [A] very far-reaching and rapid evaluation of compounds suitable for these new uses had to be carried out. This required the cooperative efforts of many industrial firms, Government laboratories, and Government-sponsored projects at universities. . . . These new products as films were admirably suited to many new uses resulting from war requirements.[12]

The instrumental role of the military in creating and perfecting these new plastics was also noted by the Quartermaster Corps itself. "Since the Army must ship and store such a wide variety of foods under adverse conditions for long periods of time, the films used for packaging must meet rather rigorous requirements. . . . Colonel Denny [from the Office of the Quartermaster General] pointed out that no one product can fulfill all of these requirements, but that the object of the Section's research is to comply with these military characteristics. He stated that recent work with Saran and thin nylon films, as well as plastic coated foils shows promise."[13]

Boyer and Dow were so eager to stake their claim that they filed a patent for "vinylidene chloride compositions stable to light" on May 4, 1945,[14] just four days after Hitler committed suicide, when the end of the war—and the restricted research program—was imminent. Saran wrap first appeared in the commercial market in 1949, as a tool for institutional and restaurant kitchens. (Ultimately, its industrial use was limited by the extremely narrow range, some twenty degrees, of its heat-seal temperature.) The final formulation, to give it flexibility while making it more impervious to heat and light, was a mix of 15 percent vinyl chloride and 85 percent vinylidene chloride with three separate plasticizers—one pound for every two of polymer. The resin was blown and then rolled to a thickness of no more than one-hundredth of a millimeter.

Four years later, Dow made its initial foray into the consumer market, introducing its new film with the advertising copy: "Only Saran-Wrap will keep it so fresh, so long . . . so easily! It clings by itself, . . . It's moisture-proof. . . . It's crystal-clear."[15] Raymond Boyer was heralded as its inventor, eventually being inducted into the Plastic Academy's Hall of Fame for his "heat and light stability studies, instrumental in the development of SARAN," and earning this line in his National Academy of Engineering biographical sketch, "[Boyer's] work with plasticizers was instrumental in the development of Saran."

On the other hand, Mark, his crew of chemists, and the Quartermaster Corps were discreetly removed from the pedigree. Said Boyer of his colleague, "Professor Mark almost deliberately tries to stay in the background where credit is concerned on any commercial matter. Hence, things like joint patents and joint publications bearing his name are virtually nonexistent. To hint at contributions would only serve to weaken existing patents which do not bear his name."[16] Zimm confirmed the self-effacement of Polytechnic and the Quartermaster Corps. "We never published any of it in the open literature. There was a big report written at the end of the project describing the things that were found. But never any papers. We found a number of things which have since been verified by other people."[17]

By the 1960s and 1970s, Saran was the leading household wrap, so much so that its trademark became the name for any clear, thin, and clingy plastic wrap, but worries over the release of chlorine gas during incineration and migration of plasticizers into food—particularly phthalate esters, the most commonly used and the dominant one in Saran—began to concern public health officials and activists. The leaching from films wasn't news to the army; in 1949 the Quartermaster Corps oversight committee on plastics had discussed "the problem of plasticizer migration and its relation to bleeding of the plasticizer onto asphalt packaging papers [a waterproof laminate of asphalt between two layers of paper],"[18] but they seemed strangely unconcerned about its inward migration into the food itself, and had gone ahead anyway. In 1997 Dow sold its Saran brand to S. C. Johnson & Son, which in 2004 discreetly changed the film's formulation to the less disintegration-prone linear low-density polyethylene (LLDPE).

★ ★ ★

KNOWING WHAT THEY—and what all chemists—knew about plastics, it appears folly that, in the early 1950s, army packaging experts proposed to find a way to heat-sterilize food and then store it for very long periods in plastic wrappers. The three materials humankind had historically used for cooking or storage vessels—ceramic, metal, and glass—soften or melt only at extremely high temperatures (a couple of thousand degrees Fahrenheit) and are either relatively inert, interacting very little with their contents, or have coatings that keep them from doing so. Not so plastic. Most common synthetic polymers used in food packaging soften at 200°F to 300°F, and as far as migration goes—suffice to say that as the molecular equivalent of a plate of spaghetti (the polymer) swimming in sauce (the plasticizer), it's easy come, easy go. It's a problem that has dogged the use of plastics in food packaging since the beginning.

In the early 1950s the Quartermaster Corps delivered a wish list to its packaging division: containers that you could manipulate in subzero temperatures, packaging for frozen foods that wouldn't disintegrate, barriers for dehydrated foods so that water vapor and oxygen couldn't penetrate them, and rations that wouldn't be the source of friendly fire wounds and casualties when air-dropped. For a while, each of these problems was worked on separately, but the solution to all quickly converged into one word: plastics. Was it possible to replace the sturdy metal cylinder, which, since the earliest days of canning, had been the favored cooking and storage vessel for moist, shelf-stable foods, with a flexible plastic pouch? In typical never-say-never fashion, the army put their heads down and got to work.

The first step was to review all the available materials and to subject them to conditions simulating that of a retort-processed ration—steam-cooking for three to fifteen minutes at 250°F, random mistreatment, and then abandonment for months. (A retort machine is an industrial canner that subjects multiple cans, jars, or pouches enclosed in a tank to high heat, in the form of hot water, spray, or steam, until their contents are sterilized.) The Quartermaster Food and Container Institute research team, led by Frank Rubinate, quickly found that the best candidate—one that wouldn't melt, harden, discolor, or disintegrate—was a combination of a layer of vinyl, a layer of aluminum foil, and a layer of polyester film. "It was really a lot of standard packaging techniques, but they had to perform at a greater level of reliability and completeness than before," explains Rauno Lampi, a food scientist who worked on the project at Natick from 1966 to 1976. "We borrowed from both the canning industry and the flexible packaging industry."

But from there, the army was stymied—it was a new technology, so to gear up, production capabilities would have to be inculcated in industry. And what better way to do that than to hold a conference, with the lure of revealing the goodies developed for the government's research program to companies that were always on the lookout for the next big thing? The attendee list read like a *Who's Who* in the American food and plastics industry: Aluminum Company of America, American Can, Beatrice Foods, Continental Can, Dow Chemical, DuPont, Eastman Kodak, Gerber Baby Foods, Goodyear Tire & Rubber Company, Kaiser Aluminum, Libby, Monsanto, Oscar Mayer, Pillsbury, Procter and Gamble, Quaker Oats, Reynolds Metals Company, Swift, Union Carbide, U.S. Industrial Chemical Company, and W. R. Grace and Company were just some of the almost sixty major corporations there.

"It should be very encouraging to the Quartermaster to realize that industry will be vitally interested, not only from a standpoint of national responsibility, but from a selfish viewpoint," commented one presenter, an equipment manufacturer, at the 1960 Conference on Flexible Packaging of Military Food Items. "Many of the food products, processes, materials and machinery which the Quartermaster requires can be used in the future by industry. The items with which he is dealing will be of great interest to the general public as items which they can consume as well as the military man."

Resolving all the technical issues—from seals that burst, processing equipment that was designed for cans, dribbly filler nozzles, and separation and migration of the adhesives used to hold together the three layers—took the army roughly two decades from the inception of the project, and resulted in innumerable innovations in the packaging industry, some of which are just now becoming industry standards, such as using ultrasound, a rapidly oscillating pressure wave, instead of heat to create seals on premade pouches. "It was a case where the objective and the momentum of the government drove all the players. . . . There were many examples of research grants coming from the Natick group into private industry to develop composite materials, the components, the equipment that actually processed these filled pouches and sterilized them. The whole system was envisioned and [then] stimulated by the government research funds," says Tom Dunn, a thirty-year flexible-packaging industry veteran and a consultant.

"But this big missing link in all of this was the adhesive to hold these individually necessary elements together into a single, synergistic packaging material," he continues. "It had to have the properties of (1) being able to withstand the high temperature and (2) being able to withstand the pressure inside the pouch, and then maintain integrity in the field with all the abuse it would encounter. While at the same time, what's not so obvious is that the overreaching concern on the part of all parties was the migration of the chemistry of these adhesives from the interface between the aluminum foil and the heat-seal layer through the food and into the food itself."

The problem of leaching of either small unattached chains of the polymer or the freewheeling plasticizers, which are liable to migrate out anyway, a tendency that increases with temperature, had been recognized by military packaging experts from the earliest days of polymer research during and immediately after World War II. With the flexible-retort-pouch project, once a set of materials had been selected, the Quartermaster Food and Container Institute commissioned outside safety studies, including one on migration of plastic components from foil-plastic laminates after high-temperature processing conditions. The research, conducted by Marcus Karel and Gerald Wogan at MIT in 1963, found that polyolefin-based laminates met FDA standards, but not those based on vinyl polymers, and that the residues from the vinyls "appeared to be aryl esters, probably phthalate." They also found that for both types of materials there were "more extractables [leached materials] from heat-sealed films."[19] The only other testing of the migration of toxins through the laminate was done by Pillsbury three years later, which concluded by calling for more studies, but basically gave the new materials a clean bill of health. Perhaps not coincidentally, Pillsbury was a member of an industry consortium led by Swift to which also belonged Reynolds Metals and Continental Can, manufacturers of the custom-designed three-ply food wrapping.

But the plastic migration problem was overshadowed by the technical challenges the Natick Center faced in turning the concept into something that could and would be produced by the food industry, and was not given another thought until 1976, when the army finally felt it could make the case to the FDA to approve the plastic food pouches for use in soldiers' rations. "Technically, we could have approved it for military use without," says Lampi. "But it would have been politically dumb not to get their approval. And that would also help the commercialization." The initial petition was rejected. The FDA was concerned about a previously unregulated carcinogen, toluene diisocyanate, a component of the adhesive. "We ran into a problem in the late [1970s] with bags intended to hold food during heating (boil-in-bags or retort pouches)," wrote an FDA official later. "At the higher temperatures, some of the laminates were insufficient barriers."[20] Meanwhile, Natick and its contractors did an end run around the adhesive issue by opting for a heat-fused laminate; the MRE with its plastic-pouch-encased entrées became standard soldier fare starting in the 1980s.

Today, the flat, plastic "flexible cans" are used widely in the Asian and European markets, but are just catching on in North America. Lampi attributes this to the deep entrenchment of the American cold chain, which moves food efficiently from factory to your fridge with nary—except for your car—an interruption in its ambient temperature of just above freezing. Dunn also points out that U.S. companies have a well-developed manufacturing infrastructure, and, unless there is a compelling reason to abandon it, will continue to use their existing equipment. But he predicts that the minute a food processor moves abroad, it will dump its old canning facilities and embrace the pouch, which is cheaper, results in better quality, and produces merchandise that can be sold to a global market, as has already happened in the shelf-stable tuna market. These products—lemon-pepper tuna, heat-and-serve fajitas, the sauce packets in frozen and ready-to-eat entrées, juice pouches—are already appearing with increasing frequency on super-market shelves.

The FDA has approved them, the market has accepted them, so now we should feel safe eating food cooked and stored in flexible pouches, right? Not so fast. Carcinogens may not have been found to leach into the food from the packaging, but that doesn't mean a lot of other things, such as the unbound monomers and plasticizers—principally phthalates, such as the ones Marcus Karel noticed back in 1963—aren't leaching into our food. The FDA's old-school toxicology still uses cancer as the gold standard: a substance triggers regulation only if it contains a known or suspected carcinogen, or is present in the food at concentrations greater than 0.5 parts per billion, a policy that was itself adopted in response to the ever-present low levels of chemicals that migrate from packaging. (This also gave rise to the exemption of well over one hundred substances, from epoxy curing agents and adhesives to antimicrobials and perchlorate, from the need for agency approval if they are present in food in those proportions.)[21]

In 2008 Congress passed and President George W. Bush signed into law the Consumer Product Safety Improvement Act, banning three phthalates—DEHP, DBP, and BBP—from children's toys. All three are used in food packaging. As part of the hearings on the issue, Norris Alderson, associate commissioner for science at the FDA, testified that "FDA-authorized uses of phthalates include uses in flexible food packaging" and, while recognizing that there was a "potential health risk," disavowed the need for regulation because "such food contact uses have been greatly reduced or eliminated through the replacement of PVC and PVDC [Saran] polymers with other polymers." His remarks concluded, "If our review indicates that existing data no longer supports the continued safe use of these materials in food contact material, FDA will take appropriate regulatory action to remove these materials from the marketplace." To date, although DEHP was banned from medical bags and tubing, no action has been taken on phthalates in food packaging. Yet in 2012 the Environmental Protection Agency (EPA) was so alarmed by the sea of phthalates in which we now live—besides food, they're found in personal care products, consumer products, toys, household dust, and soil—that it issued a Phthalates Action Plan, under the Toxic Substances Control Act, "based on one or more of the following factors: their presence in humans; persistent, bioaccumulative, and toxic (PBT) characteristics; use in consumer products; production volume." Food, according to the EPA, is the number one source of exposure.

Evidence against the plasticizer is mounting. Numerous studies, many in Asia where there is more use of polymer-packaged shelf-stable foods, have found high levels of phthalate migration into food and a high blood level of phthalate metabolites (the by-products of the body's breakdown of the ester), particularly in children. They have been shown to cause reproductive disorders in laboratory animals and are linked to endocrine disruption, such as sperm damage in men,[22] and lower IQs in children.[23] An Italian project found migration of adhesive components, including phthalates and isocyanate, the chemical the FDA was concerned about in the army's original retort pouch, in about a quarter of laminates,[24] and a recent metastudy by Korean researchers found that babies fed food from ready-to-eat plastic pouches (little brother of the MREs used for soldiers) had the highest estimated daily intake of phthalates adjusted for body weight of all subjects in the study—and that was from just one serving.[25] A diet loaded with plasticizers may be an acceptable risk for soldiers, for whom the ability to throw a squishy package into a bursting backpack and tear into it on a moment's notice is a true advantage, but maybe not for the rest of us, especially those who can't make their own choices.

★ ★ ★

ANYONE WHO'S EVER CLEANED UP A CAMPSITE knows a couple of people can generate a shocking amount of trash. That goes decuple for warriors stationed in the field and subsisting on combat rations. Each MRE contains a third of a pound of solid waste, mostly plastics and cardboard, and a recruit consumes three MREs per day; the military generates a total of thirty thousand tons of ration packaging waste annually. All of this could be recycled or turned into fuel—except for the laminated pouches, which include a foil layer and thus permanently sideline more than three million pounds of packaging material a year. Not only is the metal material unrecyclable, it adds manufacturing steps, is difficult to handle during production, is plagued by tiny ruptures, and causes problems with next-generation processing techniques. In a nutshell, foil is an expensive pain in the neck.

But the foil layer is there for a good reason. Aside from glass, which has obvious drawbacks, metal is the definitive barrier to water, oxygen, and other gases. Plastics may have smooth, shiny, and seemingly impenetrable surfaces, but in fact polymers transmit vapors; the rate at which this occurs depends on the type. For that reason, no one had ever considered an all-plastic replacement for the can. Until recently. In the late 1980s the promise of nanotechnology became a reality, making its debut in Toyota car parts. A decade later, the army decided to see if polymers filled with nanoscale particles might be an adequate substitute for the foil layer in laminated retort pouches.

To understand the world at the nanoscale (1–100 nanometers), skip the mind-boggling numbers. Just imagine human cells (10,000–30,000 nm), most of which (except for the freakish ovum) cannot be perceived by the human eye. If your cell were a house, its nanoscale contents would be about the size of appliances or smaller: a microwave-oven ribosome (25–30 nm) or a smart-phone protein (5 nm). The walls would be the cell membranes, lipid bilayers composed of stacked proteins and mobile lipids, which are porous to some hydrophobic molecules and have special protein channels or pumps—the equivalent of vents—for sugars (1 nm), amino acids (0.8 nm), nucleotides (0.9 nm), water (0.2 nm), salts, and other essential materials. Larger molecules (up to 500 nm) could enter by membrane enfolding—let's call this a door. This permeable barrier system leaves bacteria (a hulking 500–5,000 nm) out in the cold, while admitting viruses (20–400 nm). Nanoparticles, because they are so small, enter human cells more rapidly than larger particles of the same material. (This characteristic has made them a hot research topic in the pharmaceutical industry, which hopes to exploit them for drug delivery.)

Most of the nanomaterials used in food packaging are not so much designed and built but broken down—through good old-fashioned industrial processes such as milling, etching, and burning. The most commonly used (and not coincidentally the cheapest) are clays, in particular one called montmorillonite, a relation of talc, which comes in tiny platelets that are one ten-thousandth the thickness of a human hair. Because the nanoclay particles are so small, they exhibit a large surface area, which bestows special properties: better interlocking, so nanocomposites are stronger than regular materials, and more nooks and crannies—the charming technical term for this is *tortuous pathways*—so oxygen, moisture, and other gases take a really long time getting through.

In 2002, working with two of the leading providers of nanoclays, Southern Clay Products, now a subsidiary of Rockwood Specialties, and Mitsubishi's Nanocor, as well as several university contractors, Natick's own laboratory, called the Polymer Film Center of Excellence, began to patiently put through their paces various polymers and fillers. "Nanotechnology was a huge buzzword within the army," says Jo Ann Ratto, leader of Natick's Advanced Materials Engineering Team (AMET). "We even had workshops at Natick constantly involved in nanotechnology and different applications for the warfighter. So we wrote a proposal, and, because of September 11th, we ended up getting our first proposal through [very quickly]." The AMET scientists zeroed in on ethylene-co-vinyl alcohol (EVOH), a plastic that has excellent oxygen—but not moisture—resistance, is recyclable, and is considered safe by the FDA for food contact.

They tried different formulations and different ways of producing the film—cast on rollers or blown by hot air. They did detailed studies of the new plastic's structure. While the nanocomposite material was strong and had good resistance to oxygen and light, it allowed five to ten times as much water through as foil, and so was deemed inadequate to replace it—for now—in the food and retort pouches. (It also turned out to be a tasty treat for insects, so it must always be sandwiched between other layers.) But it could replace the low-density polyethylene meal bag that holds all the MRE components, using less plastic and, because of its superior moisture and oxygen resistance, allowing the items within the MRE to be more lightly wrapped.

As is ever true with the army, a setback only spurred a redoubling of efforts. The EVOH-based nanocomposite was advanced to the pilot stage and the water barrier improved by adding small amounts of another polymer, while Virginia Tech and Printpack, a major packaging company whose clients include Coca-Cola, Dole, Frito-Lay/PepsiCo, Hershey Foods, and Kraft, were contracted to review the work done so far on the new plastic and further reduce the water vapor transmission rate. (They were unsuccessful.) This only spurred a broadening of the nanotechnology net, with Natick inaugurating multiple follow-on projects. The Pliant Corporation was asked to develop a coextruded (produced all at the same time and adhered through melting) five- to seven-layer film; Appleton Coated paper company and Clemson University investigated new blending techniques (for example, one called "chaotic advection" folds two polymers together instead of mixing them, enhancing their barrier properties). Other companies worked on nanospheres, which reduce the amount of polymer needed because they incorporate air and lighten the film; bio-nanocomposites, which are made from materials such as starch, cellulose, lactic acid, and bacterial storage compounds, with the idea that these could be composted or buried; and barrier coatings. One or several of these approaches may have potential. "[The project] ended in 2012," says Ratto. "At the time, we only did it for one food item, penne pasta for retort. And now we're looking at all food items to have all-polymeric packaging. . . . I'd say in two to three years it could be in the system if performance is correct and acceptable."

However, there is much that is still unknown about nanomaterials, particularly in the areas of safety and human health. Timothy Duncan, an FDA chemist from its joint academia-government-industry Institute for Food Safety and Health, explains, "Given the number of studies that cite food packaging as a likely endpoint for PCNC [polymer/clay nano-composites] research, the number of researchers who have investigated these materials in shelf life or safety experiments using real food components is surprisingly small. . . . [While] PCNCs may represent the next revolution in food packaging technology, there are still steps that need to be taken in order to ensure that consumers are protected from any potential hazards these materials pose."[26]

As with phthalates, the FDA has not ruled on nanocomposites, instead requiring that nanoscale ingredients or additions to food-contact substances seek approval on a case-by-case base. In its June 2014 guidance for industry, only a couple of the thirty or so references addressed nanotoxicology.[27] The agency seems unlikely to take on the big—but increasingly urgent—questions anytime soon: How much do nanoscale particles migrate out of polymers? Once ingested, can nanoparticles enter living cells? Is their effect magnified many times over, as it is in inorganic substances, due to their shapes and high surface activity? Are they excreted or do they remain in tissue? And what kinds of conditions or diseases might they cause?

★ ★ ★

PROPELLED BY THE NEED to put traditional materials in service of World War II, to find cheap and plentiful substitutes for their everyday uses, and to protect rations delivered around the world in a variety of conditions, the U.S. Army encouraged the emerging field of polymer science to develop plastic food packaging, despite the obvious issues of poor temperature resistance and instability of its components. In the more than half century since Dow unleashed its—and, from behind the scenes, the Quartermaster Corps'—brainchild Saran film on the public as a way to keep food fresher, numerous other plastics have become commonplace in the supermarket and the kitchen. The Department of Defense has known since day one that plasticizers leach into adjacent materials, including food, but battlefield expediency appears to have trumped all other concerns. In the 1960s, it went ahead with an even more deterioration-prone scheme: heat sterilization and prolonged storage of food in polymer pouches. During the 1990s and early 2000s, the very period when the possible deleterious effects of the most common plasticizer, phthalates—on the endocrine system, on blood pressure, and even on IQ—were beginning to emerge, the army launched a new project exploring the replacement of the foil layer in retort pouches with nanoscale materials, although there is little to no toxicology data on the health effects of this size particle, which is perfect for entering and disrupting the human cell. In the use of plastics as food-contact substances, it may be high time we civilians abort the mission.

Chapter 11

LATE-NIGHT MUNCHIES? BREAK OUT THE THREE-YEAR-OLD PIZZA AND MONTHS-OLD GUACAMOLE

THE SACRED RITE OF TEENAGE SNACKING

I'm dreaming. Striding through a familiar city—New York, Quito, Boston? I'm free, happy, energized. (Is it a bad sign that my nightly REMs are the best part of my life?) There's a smell. Smoke. Something's burning.

"Amalia!"

I dash downstairs. A "homemade" quesadilla—presliced cheddar cheese between two flour tortillas from a plastic bag stored at room temperature—is merrily singeing in a frying pan. Strewn on the counters are other remnants of her feast, which seems to be some sort of exercise in extreme carb loading: a mostly crumbs bag of tortilla chips; a tub of ready-to-eat guacamole, a large hole carefully excavated from under its barely opened plastic film; an empty Oreo cookie tray (she has, as always, discovered her younger sisters' secret stash); and, for good measure, two dry and cold pieces of white toast. From the living room drifts the sound of canned laughter where Amalia's ensconced on the couch, simultaneously texting, Facebooking, and streaming a video on the large-screen TV. It's three o'clock in the morning.

There were times when I would have scolded her—the kitchen mess, the late hour, the poor diet, not to mention the possibility of burning down the house. But I don't. She's eighteen, home from college, fully launched along that fragile arc between childhood dependence and adult responsibility. Sometimes the best thing you can do as a parent is back off and let them grow up on their own. Besides, why sour another person's moment of happiness, short and hard-won as these are wont to be? I sigh and turn off the burner.

★ ★ ★

THE ADOLESCENT APPETITE IS NOTORIOUS. In times gone by, this meant extra helpings at meals and late-night pantry raids. Today, when most kids have their own debit cards, it often means a nonstop diet of the junkiest junk food out there, plucked from the shelves of the nearest 7-Eleven or Casey's General Store—chips, candy, frozen burritos, and that perennial favorite, pints of ice cream laden with mix-ins. But there's now hope that the teenage munchies can be assuaged in a slightly more wholesome fashion. Hurdle technology and high-pressure processing, new preservation approaches adopted or developed by the army, may aid parents in keeping their offspring cocooned in the family room, lulled with limitless quantities of ready-to-eat, room-temperature edibles—pizza, sandwiches, even guacamole and salsa. These new foods have minimal storage requirements, which means that they can be buried in closets, piled in garages, and stacked by the case in basements for months or even years. Refrigerated items can linger for months, their glowing gemstone hues almost as permanent as, well, gems.

Since humankind first figured out how to save stores for winter or for voyages over land and sea, we've understood that preservation was a devil's bargain: flavor and texture were sacrificed for staying power. Sometimes we grew to love the replacement—chewy beef jerkies, succulent hams, mouth-puckering pickles, lubricious conserves. But underlying our appreciation was the knowledge that there were no other choices. Shelf-stable food was dried, salted, sugared, pickled, fermented, or smoked. The holy grail of food preservation, juicy food that didn't rely on an abundance of salt, sugar, or acid for longevity, was unthinkable until around 1800, when Nicolas Appert discovered canning. The moist contents, cooked and stored in hermetically sealed glass or tin, revolutionized our larders. But it would be almost another two hundred years before techniques appeared that could maintain the vivid colors, honest flavors, and crisp or gooey (or both) textures of recently harvested and just-prepared foods. This special new category of edibles even has its own delightfully mind-bending adjective, "fresh-like" (mind-bending because a meaning of fresh is "not preserved").

★ ★ ★

IN THE EARLY 1960s LOTHAR LEISTNER, a scientist from the German Federal Center for Meat Research, spent a few years at Iowa State University. He apprenticed with John Ayres, an expert in the ways good food went bad, researching "the microbiology of cured meats, particularly that of ham and sausages" for the German army. He may also have been collaborating on his other specialty, mycotoxicology. According to the journal *Wissenschaft und Frieden*—a sort of German Union of Concerned Scientists, but with more humanities types—Leistner's laboratory would later develop production capabilities for four of the most lethal fungal metabolites. His publication record of the era reflects the possible dual nature of his assignment. In one journal, he describes the role of *Penicillium* in fermented sausages and, in another, its synthesis of the deadly poison ochratoxin (the latter piece was coauthored with the USDA scientist Dorothy Fennell, the Quartermaster Corps' foremost expert on fungi). Not that the fine—at times, nonexistent—line between harnessing knowledge for good or for evil should surprise anyone.

On the white-hat side of the ledger, we can probably chalk up Leistner's work to understand preservation and spoilage of traditional preserved meats: "Perhaps the first stimulation came during my research work at the Iowa State University in Ames (1963–1966), when my director, Dr. John Ayres, informed me about the work published in Australia on the importance of water activity for the preservation of food. But in my thinking, it was not only the water activity value, but the influence of several 'hurdles' which caused the preservation of foods, and thus the idea of hurdle technology slowly emerged."

Slowly indeed. It would be another decade before he breathed a word to anyone. In the meantime, Leistner continued working with Ayres, a regular contractor for the Quartermaster Food and Container Institute who often presented at conferences on yeasts and molds in preserved meats. In 1966 Leistner returned to Germany, where he "started a research project on yeasts in fermented sausages. In a way it is an extension of my work at Iowa State, but now we would like to look more closely into the correlation of yeasts to the water activity, redox potential [abbreviated Eh, the tendency to gain or lose electrons], and flavor of meats." By the 1970s he and a partner at the Federal Center for Meat Research, the microbiologist Wolfgang Rödel, were hard at work developing meat products for the German military. "The main requirements of the Germany Army were as follows: meat products should be recommended for army provisions which have fresh product characteristics and remain tasty, stable, and safe for at least 6 days at 30°C [86°F]. Refrigeration should not be required because these rations are to be used during military exercises." In 1976 Leistner, along with his colleague Rödel, published his first piece describing the concept of the hurdle effect.

It was one of those ideas that seem obvious, yet no one had come up with it before. Leistner observed that none of the steps that go into the traditional recipe for curing a porcine hindquarter would be sufficient to halt microbial infestation by itself, but together they somehow produced *prosciutto di parma, jamón serrano, Westfälischer Schinken,* or Smithfield ham, and proposed a way to explain their synergy. To understand his theory and some of the most common hurdles, let's return to the Roman Empire, which counts among its most significant achievements the spreading far and wide—if not the actual invention; that honor goes to the Celts—of the savory ham, along with Christianity, indoor plumbing, and socks. In fact, let's break down this family recipe given by Cato the Elder, a statesman and gentleman farmer, in his treatise *De Agricultura,* the earliest surviving work of Latin prose.

The first two hurdles to microbial spoilage—although, of course, it would be close to a couple millennia before we discovered microbes— would have seemed self-evident to Cato, so they are not mentioned in

his instructions. The first is chilling. In agrarian societies, hams are traditionally made in late fall and winter, when cool, but not freezing, temperatures slow microbial reproduction. After scalding, the carcass is
hung overnight, which allows blood and bodily fluids to drain and then
permits rigor mortis to set in. This brings on the second hurdle, a lowering of pH, brought about as the metabolic pathway that requires oxygen (aerobic metabolism) halts and the pathway that does not (anaerobic
metabolism) continues for a while longer, causing a buildup of lactic acid.
(In live tissue, lactic acid is regularly removed.) This increase in acidity
lowers the pH to between 4.5 and 5.6, reducing the water-binding capacity of protein so there is more "free" water to expel. Now for Cato's recipe:

> You should salt hams in the following manner, in a jar or large
> pot: When you have bought the hams cut off the hocks. Allow a
> half-modius of ground Roman salt to each ham. Spread salt on the
> bottom of the jar or pot; then lay a ham, with the skin facing
> downwards, and cover the whole with salt. Place another ham
> over it and cover in the same way, taking care that meat does not
> touch meat. Continue in the same way until all are covered. When
> you have arranged them all, spread salt above so that the meat
> shall not show, and level the whole. When they have remained five
> days in the salt remove them all with their own salt. Place at the
> bottom those which had been on top before, covering and arrang-
> ing them as before.

Hurdles three and four are all about lowering water activity through
both chemical and mechanical means. Salt diffuses into the inter- and
intracellular fluid of the meat, binding up water molecules and reducing
osmotic pressure. To maintain equilibrium, water leaches out of cells,
and eventually out of the meat. Piling the pig legs puts pressure on those
lower down, compressing tissue and pushing out additional water. A
midcycle rearrangement ensures equal treatment for all, resulting in
even more expelled water. After almost two weeks of waiting, Cato
brings us through hurdles five through seven in rapid succession.

Twelve days later take them out finally, brush off all the salt, and hang them for two days in a draught. On the third day clean them thoroughly with a sponge and rub with oil.

This hurdle—sponging clean the hams and coating them with oil—removes mold and prevents new patches from forming.

Hang them in smoke for two days—

Smoke is an antimicrobial. The cloud of hot particulate matter hovering over burning wood contains phenols, carbonyls, and organic acids, all of which alter the surface of the meat, making it more difficult for microorganisms to proliferate.

—and the third day take them down, rub with a mixture of oil and vinegar,—

Vinegar is another antimicrobial; it contains acetic acid, which kills bacteria and fungi. Oil creates a lipid barrier so new microorganisms cannot enter.

—and hang in the meat-house. No moths or worms will touch them.[1]

The final hurdle? Time. Just forget about your ham—for months. Air-drying, especially during dry and cool weather, extracts even more water, concentrates flavor, and forms a protective crust.

★ ★ ★

LEISTNER'S REALIZATION SOME TWO THOUSAND YEARS after Cato wrote his instructions that food safety and stable shelf life could be achieved by a number of mild factors working together may have been inspired by his knowledge of culinary traditions, but his theory about how the hurdle concept worked relied on the most modern microbiology. Since Van

Leeuwenhoek first spotted something wiggling under his lenses in 1675, improvements in microscopy have advanced our knowledge of cells—and the organisms made up of them—from a long shot to an extreme close-up. For the bacteria that inhabit food, this has meant a journey from Pasteur's eureka moment with the vino—"Hey! Those little critters are what's turning my Châteauneuf-du-Pape into tarnish remover"—through the decades-long toil of hundreds of bacteriologists who, like police sketch artists, pieced together elaborate profiles of the most troublesome species, to the modern-day voyeurism of microbiologists mapping out the activity of cell organelles molecule by molecule. Building on all this, Leistner articulated a new, subtler way to kill microbes. Like CIA assassins trained to elude detection, food technologists could carefully manipulate multiple low-level environmental stressors rather than rely on a single easy-to-trace murder weapon.

The reason hurdle works has to do with homeostasis, a cell's need to provide a stable environment for its inner workings. For example, temperature is vital for human cells: a few degrees up or down is the difference between life and death. Bacteria are much more forgiving with the weather, but many—although not all—are very sensitive to pH and osmotic pressure, both of which affect transport of materials in and out of the cell. Damage to the membrane alters the pumping mechanisms that maintain equilibrium, which can cause the cell to deflate or blow up. Other changes that cause irreversible harm are alterations to microbial DNA and enzymes. So-called sublethal damage is central to the hurdle technology concept. Wounded cells struggle to continue to function and to heal themselves. This depletes their energy stores, weakening them against the next assault, a process called metabolic exhaustion. Think of it as akin to shooting out your bacteria's kneecaps in a remote area—they don't die from blood loss, but from hunger and fatigue as they crawl around seeking help.

Hurdle technology also takes an ingenious approach to decimating one of the most durable life-forms on the planet, the bacterial spore, by creating a suboptimal environment—so even if it germinates, it doesn't survive for long. The outcome is like when you bring home one of those window-garden kits, plant the seeds, watch them sprout, and then forget to water them: a potful of crunchy brown tendrils. Of course, bacteria are wily buggers, and many unleash specialized survival mechanisms when confronted with a stressful environment—for example, poisonous shock proteins—or simply become even more resistant to other modes of attack. Nonetheless, the principles of hurdle technology, when managed correctly, can compensate for these virulent curveballs. As Leistner puts it:

> A synergistic effect could be achieved if the hurdles in a food hit, at the same time, different targets within the microbial cells (e.g., cell membrane, DNA, enzyme systems related to pH, a_w, Eh etc.) and thus disturb the homeostasis of the microorganisms present in several respects. If so, the repair of homeostasis as well as the activation of "stress shock proteins" become more difficult. Therefore, employing simultaneously different hurdles in the preservation of a particular food should lead to optimal stability.[2]

HOW THE NATICK CENTER HEARD about the hurdle concept remains murky. Two of the key scientists who may have had contact with Lothar Leistner or exposure to his ideas, Irwin Taub and Dan Berkowitz, have since died, leaving those on the periphery to guess. "I'm sure Dr. Taub knew of him. Whether he actually knew him and contacted him in person, I can't tell you," says Patrick Dunne, a retired Natick senior scientist. Lauren Oleksyk, the leader of the Food Processing, Engineering and Technology Team, says Berkowitz, her boss, never mentioned Leistner, and "he never called it hurdle technology." The practice itself is ancient. In the words of Michelle Richardson, the Natick food scientist with the most experience working with hurdle-based products, "If you look at the mummies, when they did the mummification, that was hurdle technology. They used chemicals, they used acids, they used several different methods to actually preserve the body." Because it's been around for such a long time, it's sometimes difficult for people to differentiate between the traditional use of the approach and its deliberate application, which includes an understanding and manipulation of the underlying biochemistry. But somehow, by the early 1990s, Natick had incorporated hurdle technology into its plans for creating microbiologically safe, shelf-stable foods.

Leistner was invited to Food Preservation 2000, a 1993 conference at the Natick Center, which assembled speakers on a host of new ideas about how to preserve food thermally and, increasingly, nonthermally. Soon after, the scientist, no slouch when it came to tooting his own horn, had the German army print up a booklet with the results of his study on "minimally processed, ready-to-eat, ambient-stable meat products for army provisions" and mailed it to five thousand food scientists and technologists around the world, to ensure that "these data became generally available." There was a snag, however. The publication was in German, an obstacle Leister was confident could be surmounted with the booklet's "many color pictures." He also began a concerted campaign to get the word out, publishing articles on the hurdle concept in *Food Research International* (1992), *Journal of Food Engineering* (1994), *Trends in Food Science & Technology* (1995), and the *International Journal of Food Microbiology* (1995).

Natick was one of the technology's earliest adopters and continues to be one of its most enthusiastic users. The Combat Feeding scientists and technologists immediately saw hurdle's usefulness to create moist items that could be stored at room temperature without loading them up with preservatives. Their first foray into hurdle technology was pound cake, but soon after that they began to work on the three-year shelf-stable sandwich, a difficult feat because the varying water contents of the different components of the sandwich tended to migrate, creating a limp and dispiriting pile. "Look at our shelf-stable sandwich; . . . for example, one of our sandwiches is pepperoni—that's a fermented product and the pH is intentionally lowered," explains Richardson. "In our bread, we have the yeast, which ferments and lowers the pH there, but in some of our formulations we actually add some acids to the bread to further lower the pH. It's not just the water activity; it's a combination of the water activity and the pH. We also add ingredients. Some of our yeasts are cured, so you have nitrite, which also has some antimicrobial activity. The packaging itself is another hurdle because it prevents moisture and gases from going inside the pouch. We put a scavenger in there, which decreases the oxygen in the headspace of the package. The organisms require oxygen, so that's a hurdle as well. We're looking at all of these together."

The shelf-stable sandwich took seventeen years from inception to its first use in rations in Iraq and Afghanistan in 2007. Gerry Darsch, the former director of the DOD Combat Feeding Directorate, explains, "We took the concept of hurdle technology and we pushed the limits . . . really ran with [it], recognizing its capacity to expand the variety and quality of products and to manage complex food matrices. . . . Most of our entrées are wet pack, but all of the shelf-stable pocket sandwiches use hurdle technology. . . . By modifying and expanding on the opportunities that hurdle technology provides, we were able to insert a whole family of products into the ration."

Hurdle can be used with all sorts of traditional food products and processes, but where it really makes a difference is with storing uncooked foods at room temperature, especially those like the army's line of sandwiches, pockets, and pizzas that have multiple ingredients of different moisture contents—dry crust, wet tomato sauce, moist cheese. In fact, the army has already developed a shelf-stable pizza—crust and sauce separated by a basil-flavored nanofilm, which should make soldiers very happy, because over the years it's been their most-requested item. On supermarket shelves, hurdle technology is everywhere—and nowhere, as most food technologists apply its principles without calling it by name. According to Kathryn Kotula, a food industry consultant who wrote a piece entitled "Interesting Forgotten Research" on hurdle technology for a food-science society newsletter, "Dr. Leistner's work is used very, very widely. So widely, in fact, that younger people probably do not know its origins."

★ ★ ★

IN A VACUUM, NO ONE HEARS YOU SCREAM (for argument's sake, we'll assume you're receiving intravenous oxygen). Without molecules to transmit sound, a wavelike disturbance of the air, it's just you, your Munchian grimace, and a vast silence. But once outside of the chamber, it's a different story. Molecules are bouncing around everywhere, responding to minute changes in temperature, concentration, mix, and volume. The force they generate and that acts on them is called pressure. Pressures can be small, like the perturbations of sound, measurable in nanopascals. (Pascal was the genius philosopher, mathematician, and scientist who insisted that vacuums do too exist.) They can be huge, such as the mammoth pressure at the center of a collapsed neutron star, estimated at from a decillion to an undecillion pascals (that's thirty-three to thirty-six zeros). Or they can be in-between; for example, a new food-preservation technique called high-pressure processing, which generally uses between three hundred million and eight hundred million pascals—imagine twenty minivans stacked on a penny—to obliterate the microbes in your edibles.

The food doesn't become a compressed inedible mass because of the magic of liquid water. In its fluid state, the molecules are about as close together as they can be at sea level (they are farther apart in ice, which is why you shouldn't forget about a bottle of wine chilling in the freezer). How does a high-pressure food-processing machine work? The food is encased in a sealed flexible package and placed inside a pressure vessel. The vessel is closed and water is pumped in until the desired pressure is obtained. The food is held at this pressure for a few minutes, generally about five, after which the vessel is decompressed and opened. (Liquid water does change volume somewhat in response to increasing external pressure, and high-moisture foods react in a similar way, compressing up to 15–20 percent. After treatment, however, the food returns to its normal volume.) In the process, some of the less powerful bonds (hydrogen, ionic, and others) break, unfolding or disassembling bigger molecules (proteins, starches, and others)—this also happens in cooking. On the other hand, the double-strength covalent bonds hold, leaving intact important smaller molecules such as vitamins, flavor compounds, and pigments. All these transformations are just fine for the food, but for the bacteria that may lurk inside, it means *finit:* cell walls spring leaks, genetic instruction manuals unravel, and their enzymes and other proteins can coagulate.

As a food-preservation technique, high-pressure processing is a late bloomer. It was discovered just before the turn of the twentieth century: in 1895, a French scientist, H. Roger, found that *E. coli, Staphylococcus aureus,* and anthrax bacteria could be killed with high pressure (although, even then, he noted that spores apparently still germinated, a problem that persists to this day);[3] four years later, Bert Hite, of West Virginia University's Agricultural Experiment Station, showed that raw milk processed with high pressure kept fresh for up to four days longer than untreated milk. While promising, research on the technique was abandoned a couple of decades later when Clarence Birdseye's invention flash freezing came along, use of which became widespread once the price of a refrigerator declined—thanks to Freon—in the 1930s. Meanwhile, the other stalwart of the modern larder, canned goods, continued to be improved, although never to the point that anyone would mistake the contents of a tin of Chicken of the Sea for a freshly seared tuna steak. Advances in knowledge and equipment for retort processing inched along, but so did the availability of high-quality fresh food. Consumers' expectations grew—and their tolerance for the mushy textures, overcooked flavors, and dull hues of canned food waned.

It was obvious that Appert's world-changing invention needed an understudy. But what? Overseen by the Quartermaster Food and Container Institute in Chicago and then the Natick Labs, the U.S. Army bet big and it bet wrong: after World War II, the government poured a scandalous number of millions of dollars into radiation sterilization, probably the biggest food research flop there ever was. In the words of Dan Farkas, an MIT-educated food scientist who spent the 1950s and 1960s as a civilian contractor on the project, "Food irradiation was the perfect case study of how not to transfer technology to the general public. There were problems at every turn. Consumers rejected it. The FDA was concerned it would be toxic. The packaging had issues." Eventually, the Natick Center's cobalt-60 irradiator was mothballed, and the scientists and engineers who'd spent a decade or more of their careers on a failed-to-launch technology were urged to find new homes—pronto. Farkas ended up at the University of Delaware.

Flummoxed about how to proceed, he did what all engineers do in times of extreme stress—he made a matrix. Across the top Farkas put all the major food-preservation techniques, and along the side, the various ways food could spoil, become poisonous, or deteriorate. He perused his table. Aha! A mechanism had been waiting quietly in a dusty corner while all the others—heat, cold, chemicals, and water activity—had had their turn. Farkas would pick up where the last scientists left off (the physicist and high-pressure expert Percy Bridgman had coagulated egg white in 1914, and a couple of small projects had been conducted in the late 1960s and early 1970s), but he would go a lot further. He would figure out a way to make high-pressure processing (HPP) commercially viable. And that would start where all good business starts, with the right equipment. Resolving this would turn out to be the biggest obstacle to converting high pressure from an impressive laboratory trick into a real alternative to thermal processing. As Farkas describes it,

> Dietrich Knorr was at the University of Delaware with me. He'd come over from Germany in the early eighties and joined the faculty, along with Dallas Hoover. The three of us decided to go into it [high-pressure processing] because we needed research dollars. . . . The only thing needed was a high-pressure unit. Parker Autoclave Engineers in Erie, Pennsylvania, made all the tubing and valves and so forth. What we would pitch to them was, that while there was a lot of interest in high-pressure metal work, it was a cyclical business—in boom times, a lot of jet engines would be built—but then . . . We suggested that the food industry would be a real . . . user of high-pressure equipment and they actually loaned us our first unit. We could roll it into the lab, hook it up, and press foods.

They spent several years figuring out the nitty-gritty, such as how much pressure and what length of time killed various bacteria in different edibles. In 1987 Farkas left for a three-year hiatus at the Campbell Soup Company, after which he moved to the University of Oregon, having been lured by a beautiful pilot plant and the chairmanship of the department. But he continued working with his University of Delaware colleagues Hoover, who was still stateside, and Knorr, who'd departed for Germany.

When the team felt that they were ready, Farkas didn't waste any time. He contacted Patrick Dunne, then a program manager at the Natick Center, whom he knew from his contracting days, his annual two-week reservist's stint in Natick's food labs, and his participation in the Natick Center's advisory board. "As soon as we saw really good microbial results at Delaware, Dallas Hoover and I took off to Natick. It seemed to be a no-brainer to go to them and show them what high pressure could do. And Dunne had a vision of taking on the new technology that could result in a better-quality food. After hearing our proposal, Pat was instrumental in building the research program that resulted in the development of [high-pressure-treated] military rations."

Taking to heart the lessons learned from the irradiation program on how not to get an exotic technology approved and adopted, Dunne got right to work. With some earmarked funds for new and novel nonthermal processes, he issued a request for a proposal under Natick's general-purpose contract vehicle, the Broad Agency Agreement, commissioning two projects: more microbiological studies at the University of Delaware and some product development work at Oregon with Farkas. By 1998 the army laboratory had concocted a very respectable all-HPP repast: seafood Creole, vegetarian pasta with tomato sauce, and yogurt with blueberries. All these foods were carefully formulated to be acidic, which made them inhospitable to most spore-forming pathogenic bacteria, including the difficult-to-eradicate botulinum, and freed them from the need for FDA approval (this is required only for "canned" low-acid and acidified foods). During the same time period, Natick moved forward on the equipment front and awarded contracts to two small companies, Avure Technologies, a spin-off from the Swedish and Swiss power and industrial machinery company ABB, and Elmhurst Research, Inc., an engineering firm, to come up with designs for machines that wouldn't, as the current ones were doing, fall apart after one hundred cycles. Durability wasn't important when the technique was used to manufacture small quantities of high-margin metal work (for example, jet engines), but for the food industry, where throughput is high and margins low, it was crucial.

The army could now kill all vegetative bacteria in acid foods and had sturdy processing equipment (the Elmhurst model recycled old six-inch cannon tubes—built to withstand powerful explosives—as the pressure vessel), but it wanted more. "We thought high pressure was pretty ripe to get expanded in the next direction," says Dunne. That direction was the elusive comfort foods—specifically, mashed potatoes—clamored for by servicemen and -women everywhere, but which until then Natick had been unable to provide, at least in a version soldiers actually enjoyed. Because the starchy side is low in acid, it must be terribly overcooked—held at high heat for a very long time—to kill any bacterial spores that could germinate during storage. Any treatment other than thermal sterilization would require regulatory approval.

ALTHOUGH FDA ACCEPTANCE had been exceedingly difficult to win for Natick's food irradiation program, Dunne was optimistic. "The task was to build this, get a shelf-stable, low-acid food, and file and get the process approved with the FDA." Taking advantage of the Dual Use Science & Technology (DUST) consortium, a new congressionally enabled DOD cooperative research vehicle that allowed government and industry to split the costs, he put together a heavy-hitting team. Avure was the prime contractor. The other companies included Hormel, Unilever, Basic American Foods, ConAgra, Baxter International, General Mills, and Mars/Masterfoods. Also part of the group was the National Center for Food Safety and Technology (NCFST, now the Institute for Food Safety and Health), a joint venture between the Illinois Institute of Technology, the food industry, and, hmm, the FDA.

The first step was to build a demonstration vessel that would use both heat and pressure for a short period—a process that came to be known as pressure-assisted thermal sterilization (PATS)—and show that it was as safe as traditional pasteurization. As anyone with a weaponizable pot–wielding great-granny knows, pressure and heat combine to drastically reduce cook time. For example, army mashed potatoes made the traditional way in a retort machine are cooked at 250°F for eighty minutes; PATS-sterilized and -preserved spuds take just twelve. It took Avure several years to successfully develop the new machines, which, at thirty-five liters, were the most capacious to date.

Then the consortium, as Dunne circumspectly puts it, "set up a [demonstration] subcontract with Illinois Institute of Technology, which happens to be a site operated by them for the FDA as the FDA's research center in food processing. They were an ideal place [to do the research], because the regulatory people who make decisions on novel processes were colocated there. . . . They are a resource [we] can bounce [off] or talk things [through] with. We [find] it important for [our] processing authority to walk steps through the research design before [we] go rather than just handing them [the FDA] a big document."

Still, HPP had no track record, minimal theoretical underpinnings, and lamentably few safety studies. The FDA's most reliable yardstick—the botulinum kill—could not be applied. To get approval for its low-acid items, the army and its collaborators would need to show that HPP and PATS were as effective as heat pasteurization, and the FDA would have to evaluate their petition using a food safety framework that permitted nontraditional sterilization techniques. In 1998 the FDA hired the Institute of Food Technologists to vet the science and safety of alternative food-processing techniques. The work on HPP was done by the Physical Processes Subpanel—three Natick contractors, Farkas, Hoover, and Jozef Kokini, a longtime army collaborator from Rutgers University—and reviewed by, among others, Dunne, staff from the NCFST, and people associated with the project, including the consultant who put together the FDA filing, Larry Keener.

Meanwhile, high-pressure processing of refrigerated acid or acidified foods was really starting to take off in the private sector. "Natick pump priming jump-started the use of high-pressure processing by food companies," says Farkas. Fresh guacamole, that most finicky and delicious dip, was the first HPP-treated food on the American market. In the late 1980s and early 1990s, Don Bowden, the owner of several Mexican restaurant chains in Texas, was looking for a way to reduce the cost and extend the life of the guacamole he served—avocados are easily bruised in shipment, and, once opened, natural enzymes quickly turn the pulp from bright green to brown. He approached Chuck Sizer, who at the time was the research manager at food packaging and processing giant Tetra Pak (he would later become director of the NCFST during the early years of its involvement with HPP). They gave thermal pasteurization a whirl. "It came back looking like pea soup," says Sizer. "The wrong color. The wrong texture. And it just didn't taste good." Eventually the pair ended up trying out the floor model at the Ohio offices of ABB.

The work of Farkas, Hoover, and Knorr earlier in the decade gave the scientist and the entrepreneur confidence. "At that time the literature was good enough to know that it had an effect on the microbiology and log reduction [the number of organisms reduced relative to the starting number] of pathogens," says Sizer. The process worked "wonderfully," leaving the avocado green, creamy, and fresh for up to a month. The new preservation technique revolutionized Bowden's business, allowing him to outsource the whole process to Mexico, and turned him, under the Wholly Guacamole trademark, into a profitable supermarket supplier. "This was the ideal product and for several years it was the poster child for high-pressure processing," says Farkas. "They just kept building plants—in Mexico, Peru, Chile. . . ."

Soon there were competitors—and new HPP products. Fresherized Foods, the company that made Wholly Guacamole, expanded its product line to avocado smoothies, salsas, and meal kits. Tropicana put a toe in the water—investing a million dollars for the exclusive rights to purchase the new HPP equipment Avure was working on for the DUST consortium,

but later withdrew because of performance issues and after initial pro-
jections suggested it wasn't cost-effective for supermarket orange juice.
However, at the opposite end of the juice market, which was inhabited
by sleek, single-portion, fresh-squeezed fruit beverages going for four or
five dollars a pop, a few companies began experimenting with the technique because it allowed them to kill dangerous microbes without flavor-
changing heat sterilization.

★ ★ ★

THE TURNING POINT IN THE ACCEPTANCE of HPP as a viable food sterilization technique came, as it so often does, after a crisis. In 1996 there had
been an *E. coli* O157:H7 outbreak that was linked to Odwalla apple juice.
Fourteen children had developed hemolytic uremic syndrome, which
destroys red blood cells, and one, a sixteen-month-old girl, died. A crim-
inal suit was filed by the FDA and multiple product liability suits were
filed on behalf of the victims. (A particularly damning piece of evidence
was a letter from the army to Odwalla rejecting it as a vendor for sanitary
deficiencies.)[4] Five years later (lengthy lag times are not uncommon for
the agency), the FDA considered, but rejected, mandating heat pasteurization for all fresh-squeezed, untreated juice, opting instead to require
that manufacturers have a Hazard Analysis and Critical Control Points
(HACCP) plan, the systems approach developed by Natick, Pillsbury,
and NASA for the space program, which is flexible about processing
methods as long as they ensure safety.

This was a major coup for Natick and its collaborators, because the
decision was based, in part, both on the DUST work being done at the
NCFST, which showed that alternative sterilization methods could be
just as effective in deactivating bacteria, and on "Kinetics of Microbial
Inactivation for Alternative Food Processing Technologies," the white
paper prepared for the FDA by the Natick-dominated IFT panel that
explained why HPP worked. The FDA's decision on fresh juice paved the
way for two important and interrelated developments: hastening a par-
adigm shift by regulatory agencies to a preventive, quality-assurance

approach to food safety rather than a reactive, inspection-based one (this was codified in the FDA's Food Safety Modernization Act of 2010), and indicating its receptivity to approving the army's new nontraditionally processed low-acid food.

The ruling also persuaded more juice makers, who were eager to preserve the just-squeezed taste without cooking the product, to turn to the new cold sterilization method. But the trickle turned into a tide in 2006, when the Hormel meat company launched the first of its Natural Choice products, a prosciutto ham; this "100% Natural. No Preservatives" line soon grew to include lunch meats, bacon, sausages, and chicken strips and is now one of the company's biggest moneymakers. (The refrigerator case is a sweet spot in terms of profitability, because the markup per item is much greater.) Other deli products manufacturers, such as Oscar Mayer, and Tyson, soon followed suit. Anchored by the investment of the meat and meat products industries, true monoliths in the American economy, the future of high-pressure processing is all but assured.

Meanwhile, the PATS consortium was finalizing its FDA filing—this was done by a knowledgeable microbiologist known as a "process authority," in this case, Larry Keener—and finishing its validation studies, which are detailed tests that show a process does what it's supposed to do under various conditions. When the consortium finally presented its petition in September 2008, FDA approval, which often goes on for years, took just five months.

This breathtaking rapidity may have been due to our ever-improving understanding of the mechanisms of microbial deactivation and that a considerable amount of scientific footwork had been done to show the technology's safety and effectiveness, but it's hard not to wonder if the fact that HPP and PATS were the pet projects of a fellow federal agency (one whose rations mandate is to seed its favored technology in the consumer market) and that the gatekeeper was also a team member played a role. Prophetically, the FDA's own Science Board had been concerned about the ethicality of exactly these types of cooperative arrangements, and discussed the topic in its October 1998 meeting:

Dr. Kipnis [professor of endocrinology]: Are there restricted limits by law as to how you can interact with this group?

Dr. Schwetz [FDA official]: No, not—for example, the two topics that I'm talking about are unrelated to a product per se; it's a new technology. So in that case, that's something that will flow through the approval systems without an awful lot of problem.

Dr. Kipnis: But new technologies are new products.

Dr. Schwetz: If it related to new products that come back to the FDA for approval, like in the Center for Devices, where we will see technologies of one kind or another, then it becomes a problem if we're helping a company develop a technology and we become one of the inventors, coming into CDRH [the Center for Devices and Radiological Health] for approval. So you're right, there are significant limits for us to be involved in this.

Dr. Nestle [professor of nutrition]: Could you tell us a little bit more about the kinds of partnerships that you're seeking, because I'm very concerned about the potential for conflict of interest here. I just can't think of anything that wouldn't be a conflict of interest.[5]

Everything seems to have been done by the book, but there's an unnerving circularity to the arrangement. So far, there's no evidence that consumer health has been put at risk, although human safety studies on the new food-processing techniques are still scant. At any rate, the outcome was that just about any food—including meat, poultry, and eggs, the USDA's domain—can now be high-pressure-processed. Gerry Darsch sums it up: "If we don't get industry on board, particularly if it's something relatively novel, it's not going anywhere. We don't want something military-specific." And should you have any lingering doubts about whose baby this really is, the Natick Center's recently retired Pat Dunne doesn't. "Where I personally really made the market commercially—it's refrigerated, extended-shelf-life foods."

Chapter 12

SUPERMARKET TOUR

T he Natick Center's tentacles not only grasp the items we examined from our children's lunch boxes, they're everywhere in the American food system. So let's go to the supermarket. My local Star Market is down at the heels, feeling the pressure of the Trader Joe's and Whole Foods less than a mile away, although the parking lot is usually full. The shoppers give off a watching-every-last-penny vibe. I usually come here after I've dropped off my youngest daughter for gymnastics practice, so I can stock up on cheap packaged and convenience foods. Today is different, though. Instead of shopping for my family, I'll fill my cart with every item I can identify* that has a military provenance or influence.

Our first stop is right next to the entrance: the produce section. The rainbow heaps of fruits and vegetables in bins in the middle of the floor are close to their natural state, but if we stroll along the periphery, there are lots of items with a military link. I always toss in a bag or two of prewashed salad—there's nothing easier than tearing one open and

---

* There are certainly many more. Researching these foods' scientific and technological pasts as well as those of items that have no apparent U.S. Army connection would undoubtedly uncover an even broader military impact.

dousing the contents with dressing, right? The modified- or controlled-atmosphere packaging systems are an outgrowth of army research into keeping FF&V (the industry abbreviation for fresh fruits and vegetables) in good condition during shipment and storage. In the 1950s the U.S. Navy was among the first to use polyethylene bags to increase the shelf life of produce; by controlling oxygen and carbon dioxide levels, they slowed its respiration, delaying ripening and spoilage. In the 1960s the Quartermaster Corps, working with the appliance manufacturer Whirlpool, began to experiment with a modified-atmosphere container, which replaced the natural atmosphere with a custom blend of gases that helped extend shelf life. The first experiments involved fresh lettuce and celery shipped to Vietnam during the war. In the 1980s this expiration-date-extending tool began being used routinely for individual consumer articles, and it is now, according to the packaging expert Aaron Brody, the food innovation with the greatest impact—at least if measured by the number of supermarket perishables that use it to maintain freshness. In 2005 Fresh Express, an outgrowth of the original Whirlpool project that controls 40 percent of the packaged salad market, was bought by Chiquita Brands International for $855 million.

Nearby are a couple cooler cases of fresh-squeezed juices and smoothies, many of them cold-pasteurized with high-pressure processing, one of several new sterilization techniques spearheaded by the army. Odwalla, the original, is fighting off incursions by newer brands such as Naked Juice (a subsidiary of PepsiCo), Suja, Evolution Fresh (Starbucks), and BluePrint (Hain Celestial Group). The big, pricey bottles have names like Easy Greens, Defense Up, Green Machine, and Protein Zone, all staking their claim—unproven—to a salutary effect on your body. Same deal for that array of chilled prepared guacamoles and salsas. In fact, even that forlorn little display of serving-size bags of ready-to-eat cut fruits and vegetables relies on the new processing technique: Bites, Chiquita's packaged apple slices and carrots, and Reichel Foods' Dippin' Stix, which combine about half an apple's worth of slices or a handful of carrot sticks with a tub of high-pressure-processed caramel sauce or ranch dressing. No one's lining up for these, though; I guess they haven't caught on yet.

The next section, prepared foods, seems to be an unspoken answer to your daily what's-for-dinner quandary. How about making your "own" pizza? That rack of red-and-green-plastic-encased Boboli crusts never stales thanks to hurdle technology; the same goes for the flatbread and the soft room-temperature tortillas. Or, look over there: heat-'n'-serve meals—short ribs, chicken parmesan, mac 'n' cheese—just ready to pop in the microwave. Which has a military origin, of course.

The microwave oven is a descendant of the magnetron, an electromagnetic oscillator that made radar much more efficient by reducing the size of the equipment so that it could be installed on ships and in submarines. The devices were produced by the longtime defense contractor Raytheon. An apocryphal story is told about the appliance's invention: One day in 1945 a technician testing the equipment found that his chocolate bar had melted. The Quartermaster Corps immediately seized on the idea as a way to "defrost and heat a pre-cooked meal in one minute. . . . Of foremost importance will be the problem of feeding heavy bombers' crews likely to be traveling for 10,000 miles,"[1] and helped to fund the development of the microwave oven. Licensing the technology a decade later, the stove manufacturer Tappan (now part of Electrolux), and appliance giant Westinghouse produced the first ridiculously expensive—$2,000 to $3,000 (in 1950s dollars)—and clunky wall-mounted machines. Eventually, after the price and size came down and the public got comfortable with the concept, the ovens became standard kitchen gear.

Here we are at the meat department. I usually get a couple of packages of something mild-flavored and quick-cooking: chicken breasts, sirloin strips, every now and then a pork tenderloin that I make in the toaster oven. The Natick Center owns this section; its handprints are so numerous it's hard to begin. I see boneless meat shipped in boxes and restructured meat products, which line the deli and freezer cases and— stepping outside the grocery store for just a moment—the walk-ins of fast-food restaurants. The army even had a role in developing the process for eviscerating the poultry that goes into your favorite cutlets, patties, and nuggets. And let's not forget high-pressure processing; because it sterilizes with little or no cooking, it allows you to enjoy your favorite heat-'n'-serve precooked entrées—fish, chicken, beef—as well as additive-free deli meats.

A little farther along is the wall of refrigerators housing an array of dairy products. We can bypass the traditional cheeses and pasteurized milk, but we can thank the military for helping to spread the acceptance and use of processed cheese far and wide with an assist from its longtime collaborator Kraft; for developing lactose-free powdered milk with the USDA; and for figuring out how to sterilize, stabilize, and extend the life of egg products. I'm still on the perimeter of the supermarket, however, where nutritionists say the healthy, "unprocessed" food resides. It's time to venture into the hinterlands, the dozen or so aisles glutted with packaged room-temperature foods, many of which owe their existence to the food science funded or supported by Natick in its never-ending quest to provide durable rations that can survive unrefrigerated for years in a range of climates.

Let's hit the bakery section first, where way back when, the army helped to develop active dry yeast; then funded the trial runs for bacterial enzyme–softened bread; and, most recently, figured out how to forestall staling with humectants and starch recrystallization inhibitors. Another major war-related contribution to the supermarket loaf is enrichment, which dates to the early 1940s, a time when diseases and conditions such as goiters, pellagra, beriberi, and anemia, all caused by dietary deficiencies, were common, and the service branches were forced to reject almost half of the first two million war recruits for health issues related to malnourishment or poor medical care. To address this shocking deficiency, President Roosevelt convened a National Nutrition Conference for Defense. At the May 1941 meeting, which was attended by more than eight hundred people, it was decided to develop a universal rubric for daily caloric, nutrient, vitamin, and mineral needs. The task was given to the Committee on Food and Nutrition, whose work eventually led to the founding of the bread enrichment* program, which mandates the addition of B vitamins to all commercial loaves.

For those who prefer the joy of homemade baked goods but just don't have the time—and who does?—the Quartermaster Food and Container Institute developed all kinds of mixes, from cakes to quick breads, in the 1950s. In fact, one of the brand names most associated with housewifery, Betty Crocker, has been a major beneficiary of military technology; the easy meals in its latest product line, such as carne asada, garlic chicken, and beans, come in retort pouches. Why, it's even started selling shelf-stable mashed potatoes, the army's first low-acid pressure-assisted thermal sterilization (PATS) food. The mother lode of military influence is the ready-to-eat staples of dorm rooms, offices, and, increasingly, because you are, of course, "crazy busy," your larder. Breakfast pastries. Energy bars. Big, toothy chocolate chip cookies. All of them are intermediate-moisture foods, often a packaged bakery treat or one that has a baked component with a soft and chewy texture.

I stop at the end of a middle row for a moment to stare at what appears to be a commemorative display of old C rations. Here, almost as if they were deliberately assembled, are the consumer versions of World War II soldier food: Underwood's Deviled Ham Spread, Hormel's Dinty Moore Beef Stew and Spam, Swift's Vienna Sausage and dried chipped beef in all its glory. I pause for a moment to pay homage to the technology that began it all, first promulgated by Napoleon and relied on in most of the American wars fought in the late nineteenth and twentieth centuries. (On another occasion, as part of my research, I brought home some to try. Reactions were mixed. The kids said the deviled ham looked like cat food and ran shrieking from the room. My husband waved away my proffered Vienna sausage with "Sometimes we had to eat those in Cuba." My mother, on the other hand, polished off her plate of chipped beef on toast, although she said, with a sigh, "My mother's cream sauce was thicker.") As I continue walking down the aisle, the cans come in

---

* The difference between enrichment and fortification is that enrichment returns vitamins and minerals lost in processing, while fortification adds new ones.

waves organized by food type: soups, fruits, vegetables, beans. Finally the shiny cylinders give way to rows of plastic-and-foil-laminated retort pouches—the culmination of almost two decades of army and contractor work, including an Institute of Food Technologists prizewinning collaboration between the Natick Center, Reynolds Metals, and Continental Can. Here I find items such as tuna, pet food, rice dishes, heat-'n'-serve entrées and sides, sauce packets, juice pouches, and squeeze yogurts. Campbell's is obviously seeking a younger, hipper market with its new pouched Go Soups; black-and-white portraits of "real people" grace the Chicken & Quinoa with Poblano Chilies and Moroccan Style Chicken with Chickpeas.

Blink and you'll miss the display of cinnamon, pepper, and marjoram in little glass or plastic bottles—the greatest scientific breakthrough ever, the splitting of the atom and the harnessing of the tremendous energy that generated the atomic bomb, relegated to the spice rack. After the Manhattan Project, which had employed 130,000 people for four years straight with an investment of $2 billion ($26 billion in current dollars), was shuttered at the end of 1946, the United States was left with a network of nuclear reactors. So the army and the Atomic Energy Commission (AEC) began experiments with the application of gamma rays (electromagnetic waves considerably shorter than the diameter of an atom) to sterilize food. Because very little escapes their tiny wavelength, bombarding anything with gamma rays is guaranteed to kill what hides inside, including bacteria and their almost indestructible spores. The Manhattan Project's spent fuel assemblies, which still emitted "quite deadly" gamma rays, according to Charles Horner,[2] an AEC official, were recycled into food irradiation facilities constructed around the country, the first in Dugway, Utah.

The Quartermaster Corps' radiation sterilization project, which a few years after it began received the ringing endorsement of President Eisenhower as part of the Atoms for Peace program, would eventually cost the U.S. taxpayer $80 million. By the mid-1950s it had an enormous cast from government, academia, and business, including the Atomic

Energy Commission, the USDA, Swift, General Electric, the American Meat Institute, and dozens of universities—a list that would over time number more than 120 institutions.[3] MIT's participation was led by Bernard Proctor, who had managed the Subsistence Research Laboratory's outside research programs during World War II.

From the start, the food irradiation program was plagued by problems. The energy of the beams left in their wake all sorts of chemical reactions: many deteriorated the food's flavor, texture, and nutritional quality; others seemed to create new substances called unique radiolytic products, about which little was known. Despite the Natick Center's assurance that it "would not induce radioactivity in the foods, above the background level,"[4] the public was wary. Why, if a nuclear explosion was so devastating to human life and health, would we use atomic energy on our food? The army was forced to undertake numerous health and safety studies; in fact, it's said that effects of food irradiation have been scrutinized more than any other food technology. Then the 1958 Food Additives Amendment to the Food, Drug, and Cosmetic Act defined a source of radiation as a food additive, which triggered regulation by the FDA.

By the early 1960s although Natick had made great strides in both figuring out how to maintain palatability by excluding oxygen from the environment and using heat to deactivate enzymes before processing, the army was having second thoughts about using radiation to sterilize food, doubting its cost-effectiveness. Around the same time, a study by a trio of Cornell scientists on the use of irradiated nutrient sources—coconut milk, which offers an exceptional growth medium, for carrot plants and sugar for fruit flies—found that they induced genetic mutations. These two developments attracted the attention of the press and brought an onslaught of articles about the effects of eating radiation-sterilized food. Despite this, the FDA felt convinced that at least low-dose treatment was safe, and approved it for disinfecting wheat and preventing sprouting of potatoes. Confident that approval of irradiated meat was just around the corner, Allen Products Company (a manufacturer of optical equipment), Martin Marietta (a heavy building materials supplier), and Uniroyal (a tire company) began to plan a radiation sterilization facility large enough to satisfy both military demand and—they hoped—the new commercial market.

Those hopes were dashed in 1968, when, after requesting and reviewing additional DOD-sponsored studies that seemed to show drops in fecundity and increases in stillbirths in rats and dogs fed irradiated meat, the FDA denied the Defense Department's petition to radappertize (their term, combining *radiation* with *appertize,* in honor of Nicolas Appert) ham. At the same time, the agency also rescinded the approval for canned bacon it had issued in 1963. The army was not deterred. "The Committee on Radiation Preservation of Food, in Executive Session, unanimously and forcibly recommended that the Army Food Irradiation Program be continued and funded at the level needed to result in the issuance of regulations for at least four foods . . . [:] ham, chicken, beef and pork."[5] To ease the way, the committee proposed that the National Academy of Sciences–National Research Council (NAS-NRC) be charged with undertaking a review of all the safety studies of irradiated food and set criteria for its wholesomeness "to assist regulatory agencies in the U.S. and elsewhere whose responsibility is to approve to use of irradiated foods for human consumption."

A new set of studies was done by Natick under the oversight of NAS-NRC and "in close cooperation with the FDA," and in the early and mid-1970s reports were issued declaring irradiated food to be "toxicologically safe." In 1984 the FDA approved low-dose radiation sterilization of fruits and vegetables, which allows importers to omit lengthy and expensive quarantines, and high-dose radiation sterilization of spices. A full thirteen years later, the FDA finally approved radiation sterilization of meat, which can be done with not only gamma rays but also electron beams and X-rays, and many other foodstuffs. But although these products finally made their commercial debut in 1997, they were never widely accepted by consumers.

Down the same aisle are some familiar foods made with a military technology that had a bit more traction than food irradiation, but not much. Instant coffee, instant soup, powdered beverages, the little nibs of fruit in cereals, and the vegetables and herbs in flavoring packets for rices and pilafs are descendants of the freeze-dried blood products and vaccines delivered to battlefield medics during World War II. The industry that "grew almost spontaneously under the stimulus of either patriotic duty or adventurous speculation" foundered in the 1950s, however, with most firms going bankrupt.[6] The armed forces persevered, but finally, after decades of research, closed the chapter on freeze-drying, restricting its use to extreme situations, such as Arctic expeditions and long-range patrols, where reduced weight is imperative and appetites are honed by exertion and deprivation. Nonetheless, in their work on the project, Natick-funded scientists made important breakthroughs that have contributed greatly to other areas of food science; for example, prediction and control of water activity, nonenzymatic browning, and lipid oxidation.

Before I leave the pantry staples, I grab a box of converted rice, which has been parboiled so that the starch absorbs many vitamins and minerals, then hulled to make it more palatable to consumers. First served to soldiers during World War II, the grain was the brainchild of Eric Huzenlaub, an English chemist who had labored for ten years to perfect the process (used for centuries in India), but failed to bring it to market. It would have died on the vine but for a plucky proposal by Gordon Harwell, an aspiring American entrepreneur, who shamelessly hounded the Quartermaster Corps brass, waving a copy of a University of Arkansas study that found converted rice kept its nutrients and imploring them to give him a chance. By the end of the war, the two partners' plant in Houston, Texas, was humming, as were four more throughout the South. "The new rice was classified by Col. Rohland A. Isker, research director of the Quartermaster Corps, as one of the most significant scientific developments of World War II."[7]

Detouring into the freezer section for the armload of frozen pizzas at which my children now glare mutinously when I bring them home, I pass the TV dinners. Turns out Swanson was the second manufacturer of the reheatable meals; the first was an army contractor, Maxson Food Systems, which invented Strato-Plates—meat, vegetables, and potatoes frozen in a tray—to serve to troops on overseas flights. A few steps down from the frozen dinners are cans of orange juice concentrate. Starting in 1942, a team of USDA food scientists in Florida worked feverishly to invent a method to reduce the water content of orange juice but still leave it tasting like just-squeezed fruit to ensure that troops got enough vitamin C; their low-temperature evaporation process, which reduced water by 80 percent, was perfected as the war ended in 1945, just in time for the Quartermaster Corps to place its first order with a supplier—and cancel it. The company quickly revamped the product as a consumer convenience food, Minute Maid frozen concentrate.

It's a good thing I lift weights; my cart is getting awfully heavy, but we can't leave before visiting the laundry, paper, and cleaning product aisle. Bet you didn't know the army has had an outsize impact on the way you store, prepare, and clean up food at home. For example, almost every appliance in your modern-day kitchen has a military lineage. We already covered the microwave, but the army also had a hand in the development of safe coolants for refrigerators, although their interest was primarily in preventing fires in aircraft engines. Chlorofluorocarbons (CFCs) were originally hailed as an alternative to explosion-prone ammonia-based refrigeration systems—their destructive effect on the ozone layer was discovered much later. (And it would be remiss not to mention the War Department's invention of aerosol sprays, which originally expelled not cheese sauce or whipped cream but CFCs as an insect repellent.) Dishwashers, although invented by Josephine Cochrane, a socialite, in the late 1800s—the originals were hand-cranked—were the realm of restaurant and institutional but not home kitchens until the Quartermaster Corps redesigned them during World War II and afterward, making them cheaper and more efficient, to prevent the transmission of food-borne illness in mess halls. In addition, the military sponsored the study and improvement of no-rinse detergents and other cookware cleaners. Or, for those who'd rather omit the cleanup and eat picnic-style, you can thank the army for laminated paper plates and plastic forks, spoons, and knives. And after the meal is done, store the leftovers in cling wrap, now mostly made from linear low-density polyethylene instead of vinylidene chloride like the original Saran, or aluminum foil, which entered the consumer market after the Surplus War Properties "cannibalized" World War II's 150,000 surplus combat planes—that's more than fifteen times the number of U.S. commercial aircraft flying today[8]— by melting them down into aluminum ingot, a cheap raw material that Reynolds and other tin companies then turned, for the first time, into a foil for home use.

And finally, I shouldn't forget what, by law, must be printed on every box, bottle, or bag: nutritional information. World War II was the first time the diet of soldiers in the field differed dramatically from that of civilians, being composed almost entirely of rations made from processed foods. Not only did the army struggle with the issue of palatability and monotony, which sharply affected the caloric intake of recruits, but by necessity it was forced to ask the questions: Is this diet equivalent to home-cooked food? Does it have the right types and amounts of nutrients for optimal health? Until then, the Surgeon General of the Army had dictated the contents of rations, basing his guidelines on what was considered to be a healthful diet: so many portions each of fresh or salted meat, peas or beans, fresh and dried fruits and vegetables, grains, and hardtack or fresh bread. Faced with the new canned or packaged C, D, and K rations, this was no longer feasible. As part of its extensive wartime research and development program, the army first reviewed the available literature, studied in its own labs and those of its university and industry contractors, and then determined the exact set of nutrients— chemical substances such as proteins, fats, carbohydrates, minerals, and vitamins—that were required to maintain health. In the intervening years, these have been updated many times, with new information provided by government agencies, medical researchers, and nutritionists. This shift, though it seems slight, had monumental consequences: thinking in terms of nutrients, rather than foodstuffs, allowed people to divorce the concept of a good diet from eating foods in their natural state and believe that this could, at least in theory, be achieved by consuming the allotted RDAs from processed foods.

I push my overflowing cart to register 7, which is operated by an old man wearing the garish store uniform of bright blue polyester shirt and black vest. His back is so bent his nose practically rubs the scanning machine. There on the impulse display rack are a few more items. M&M's, Mars's iconic candy, was invented just in the nick of time to be under exclusive contract to the U.S. military during World War II—there was no need to advertise when sixteen million soldiers returned home craving the "chocolate that melts in your mouth, not in your hand," and Wrigley's gum, another 1940s ration add-in, received a permanent upward bump in market position. Or to tempt the salt-loving, bags of Frito-Lay's Cheetos or other cheesy snack foods made from surplus cheese powder, or tubes of perfectly shaped Pringles chips made from dehydrated potatoes, a 1950s army project with the USDA.

Beep. Beep. Beep. My cashier slowly but steadily runs my items past the laser scanner. He stops for a moment, and his white eyebrows shoot up quizzically, his magnified gray eyes suddenly alert. He waves my six-pack of 21st Amendment Brewery's Bitter American beer at me, pointing to the chimpanzee in a space suit that's drawn on the carton. "Do you know where that's from?" he demands, obviously prepared to tell me.

"Yes. That's Ham, the chimp that was sent into space just before the first manned Mercury flight in 1961." He looks surprised, then impressed. It's on the tip of my tongue to go on. I think, "Actually, my cart is full of combat rations and astronaut food. The technology that went into producing them is here in my instant coffee, in my package of granola bars, in the 'all natural' minimally processed packaged pastrami." But instead I bite my tongue—hard. Lately, I've started to teeter precariously on the line between fun-fact-filled friend and deadly dinner pundit. Like an anger management graduate, I've had to learn to recognize my triggers. And one of mine is that treacherous little corrective "actually."

★ ★ ★

OF COURSE, my overladen shopping cart contains only the military influence on our food system that you can see, touch, and taste. There are many others that affect everything from transportation and storage to government policy and programs, to food research and marketing, and more.

The military has had a decisive hand in many of the innovations that form the modern-day distribution system. Although it did not invent the ISO (International Standards Organization) container in which all the world's goods are now shipped, it gave the then-radical concept of a steel box that could move from truck bed to train to ship without being loaded and unloaded the major boost it needed to enter and dominate the market by adapting it for all DOD shipments starting in the early 1970s. The efficiency gained from using containers reduced shipping costs by a stunning 90 percent. Inside the container, the standard-size four-way pallet placed by a forklift is another invention that owes its existence to military ingenuity during World War II. Vastly improved corrugated fiberboard boxes, another material-handling staple, was a long-term cooperative project between the Quartermaster Corps and Forest Products Laboratory, a Wisconsin-based USDA research lab that develops new or better industrial uses for wood. Their design for boxes able to withstand high pressure, stress, and moisture was disseminated in the public realm during the 1950s, free for use by any takers.

One of the military's most important unseen contributions is to food safety, through the internationally accepted protocol for reducing contamination risks, Hazard Analysis and Critical Control Points (HACCP). The system was invented during the Space Race—because if there's a time you definitely don't want to be felled by stomach cramps, nausea, vomiting, diarrhea, or worse, it's hurtling at 17,500 mph in a tiny capsule with two other human beings. NASA set its sights high, adopting a "zero-defect" acceptance policy for astronaut provisions. Remembered the biologist and nutritionist Paul Lachance, a project leader for NASA, "The U.S. Army had already dabbled in this field, and they, as a matter of fact, had developed a document, which I don't know the name of, but they had a document for a procedure for trying to minimize military feeding contamination."[9] This was the Natick Center's "modes of failure," a system for ensuring the safety of medical supplies. Using the army's approach as a model and the safety standards developed in its laboratories, Quartermaster Corps contractor Pillsbury, led by the microbiologist Howard Bauman; Natick; and NASA came up with HACCP, a seven-point plan that begins with an inventory of the food manufacturing process, from raw material to finished product, and identifies all the junctures at which microbiological contamination could occur. A protocol is then set up, with careful record making of measurements at all the control points and limits beyond which corrective action is required. Spontaneous and long-term monitoring of this data allows managers to control the quality of their products and government officials to verify that the procedure is working correctly.

Pillsbury and other space program food suppliers were required to use this system for astronaut provisions. Then, in the early 1970s, some of Pillsbury's baby cereal was found to be laced with glass, and another company had a high-profile case of botulism-infested vichyssoise soup. At that time, some businesses began to spontaneously implement the HACCP principles, including fast-food giant Burger King. Finally, by the 1990s, after the public was outraged by sales of *E. coli*–laced hamburger meat, the USDA began to require that meat companies have HACCP plans in place. They were followed in the early years of the 2000s with similar regulations by the FDA for fresh juice, mollusks, and alternatively processed foods. In 2011 President Obama signed into law the Food Safety Modernization Act, which, among other measures, for the first time required that all food facilities have in place an HACCP plan.

In war, even with the tastiest rations, fighters tend to lose weight and become dehydrated. Exactly why, after seventy-five years of army research, is still not clear, although the military is a lot better at getting recruits to consume enough calories and nutrients and to stay hydrated. But in seeking to understand the reasons people like and eat one food and not another, the military ended up creating a brand-new field: food acceptance research, which includes the conceptual frameworks and instruments that are standard in the food industry to this day.

The work began during World War II, with the investigations of the National Research Council's Committee on Food Habits, a wartime group headed by, among others, the legendary cultural anthropologist Margaret Mead. Its purpose was to figure out how to persuade people to change their eating habits—vital for consumers when rationing made familiar foods unavailable and unfamiliar ones had to be substituted, as well as for soldiers who would be subsisting on diets unlike those they followed at home. Explained Mead, "It is also necessary to know . . . how changes may be phrased so that they will be accepted and welcomed, what phrases should be avoided because they will awaken anxiety, mere temporary compliance, or actual resistance."[10] (The specific task with which the committee was entrusted was persuading the American public to eat organ meat.) Over the course of its five-year existence the Committee on Food Habits undertook, funded, or endorsed more than two hundred studies. In 1945 this function was absorbed by the Quartermaster Food and Container Institute, with the founding of the Food Acceptance Laboratory under the supervision of W. Franklin Dove, a biologist who'd done some work on human preferences. One of its earliest endeavors was collecting, through university partners, data on regional likes and dislikes and compiling a master list of national favorite foods. (Apparently hamburger had a surprisingly strong showing; this may have inspired the founders of the first fast-food restaurants.) The investigation was done using paired preferences—choosing which item of two was liked best—and it became the modus operandi of army food research thereafter.

One of the most enduring and important contributions of the Food Acceptance Laboratory was the development, with the University of Chicago, of the nine-point hedonic scale as a way to measure consumers' reactions to foods. In the instrument, the numbers one through nine correspond to reactions from extreme dislike to extreme liking; it was found the longer scale helped ferret out small but significant differences in overall appeal. Because it's so easy to use and understand, it has become the standard worldwide. The importance of the Quartermaster Corps' work on food acceptance research can be judged by the number of its alumni who went on to lead food acceptance research in private industry, including at companies such as Coca-Cola, Pillsbury, Lipton,

ConAgra's Hunt-Wesson, Ocean Spray, and Pizza Hut, as well as numerous Natick Lab graduates who found places in other government agencies and academia.

★ ★ ★

LOOK BEHIND ME. If we removed every item with an army origin or influence, any grocery store would be at least half empty.* Now do you see how the military's stranglehold on basic food science and technology research means that the Combat Feeding Program's decisions about how to feed warfighters become de facto decisions about how to feed you?

---

* At the end of the interviews I conducted for this book, I asked subjects to estimate the percentage of products in the supermarket with a military origin or influence. None felt they were expert enough on the subject to be quoted, but their guesses ranged from 30 percent to 70 percent.

Chapter 13

COMING UP NEXT FROM THE HOUSE OF GI JOE

They have chiseled chins, keen eyes, gleaming teeth, and impeccable haircuts. Depending on their specialty, they might be bespoke-suited, button-down and khaki-clad, or supercasual in jeans and an edgy shirt. Their speech is peppered with terms like IPO, Series A, burn rate, and M&A. And their net worths—let's just say healthy. Venture capitalists live at the intersection of macho and money, and they like their companies as fast and risky as the Porsches they inevitably drive.

Businesspeople often reserve their greatest scorn for the idea of government funding of innovation. Inept. Plodding. Unprofitable. "Let the market choose!" they say. In this they assault their own bloodline. Venture capitalism, which began in the years immediately following World War II, seeks to find entrepreneurs with great ideas or embryonic companies with game-changing inventions. Then, in exchange for shares, it supplies them with enough money to get through the difficult period while their products (they hope) gain traction in the marketplace. The final step is to sell the successful enterprises to larger businesses or invite in investors, filling everyone's coffers in the process. This approach is directly inherited from Georges Doriot, the "Father of Venture Capitalism," who cut his cash cowboy teeth developing better equipment and supplies for the Quartermaster Corps. He then went on to found the firm American Research and Development Corporation (ARDC), which, among other things, shepherded the enormously successful computer manufacturer Digital Equipment Company, itself built on the army's early and deep research in information technology, from a start-up to a behemoth—a five-hundred-fold return on initial investment. (Electronics, another heavily military-supported field, became ARDC's other technology sweet spot.) The business journalist Spencer Ante summarizes Doriot's approach in *Creative Capital:*

> When Doriot became head of the Military Planning Division in the Office of the Quartermaster General, he began running, in a sense, his first venture capital operation. The purpose of his division was to identify the unmet needs of soldiers and oversee the development of new products to fill those needs. In order to pull off this engineering miracle, Doriot perfected the art of finding the right people for the right technical challenge, and then inspiring them to invent the future. [1]

The wartime Office of Scientific Research and Development (OSRD), headed by the former MIT dean and Carnegie Institute president Vannevar Bush, faced staggering scientific and technological challenges, from creating the first atomic bomb and developing synthetic rubber to studying the physiological effects of starvation (research conducted by Ancel Keys, inventor of the K ration). Much of this work was done by universities, industry collaborators, and government laboratories. At first from necessity, and then probably because it worked, OSRD funded multiple organizations to take on the identical or closely related aspects of the same problem, helped them to resolve issues when they arose, and, at the end, winnowed the choices to one or a few approaches. Doriot, whose Quartermaster Corps assignment fell under the agency's umbrella, would certainly have followed suit.

This system—championed, if not invented, by Doriot—is used every day in modern venture capital firms when they review the field, do due diligence, and select a couple of strong prospects; provide financial, managerial, and technical support; oversee and assist leading players; and—the prize!—sell the successes or take them public. It's also the standard operating procedure for DOD research endeavors, one handed down intact through generations of military technocrats. There are, however, some crucial differences between public and private sector methods. The government focuses on basic or early-stage applied research or on the development of technology that, at that moment, has a clear military purpose but not necessarily a consumer one. To best support fledgling efforts, the armed forces finances specific research or projects, is relatively unconcerned about marketability, and is willing to support work over a longer time frame. Goal: functionality. Venture capitalism comes in after the developmental heavy lifting has been done and provides enough financing to fine-tune the product, run the business for a short to medium time frame, and push it into the marketplace. Goal: profitability.

In point of fact, military and government funding of research and venture capitalist support of new technology firms are deeply complementary. This innovation one-two has already happened in computing, communications, and electronics, where after the science and technology infrastructure was laid by the army, businesses sprouted and prospered. And allowed you, the consumer, to enjoy computers, the Internet, jet planes, wireless communications, smartphones, global positioning technology, and much more. The venture capitalist who wants to know where the growth areas of tomorrow will be should watch where the military puts its money today—both because its investment likely signals the presence of an undeveloped or underdeveloped technology sector and because the approaches it knights are more apt to prevail, a nexus that spells earnings. As Doriot's partner in ARDC, the renowned financier Merrill Griswold, pointed out, "venture capital [is] most successful where it [is] able to pioneer new economic spaces."[2]

Of course, Doriot wasn't the only one to apply wartime knowledge and skill to peacetime moneymaking. Less well-known former Quartermaster Corps subsistence research staff also turned their World War II experiences into business enterprises, as owners, investors, or executives. MIT's Bernard Proctor returned to Cambridge to oversee the army food irradiation program; he also took out a patent on the equipment, should it ever be commercialized, and bought stock in a number of military food research–related ventures, including potato dehydration, condensed milk, orange juice, and soda. In fact, he helped the company Cantrell & Cochrane iron the kinks out of a revolutionary new product: a highly corrosive, pressurized liquid in a tin cylinder, aka canned soda.[3] Another alumnus who profited from his army ration research experience was the biochemist George Gelman, the first director of the Quartermaster Food and Container Institute for the Armed Forces; shortly after leaving the service, he cofounded with Jerry Sudarsky the California company Bioferm, a producer of vitamin B_{12}, insecticides, and monosodium glutamate (MSG), which was later acquired by International Minerals and Chemical. "George Gelman . . . is a millionaire today,"[4] recounted Emil Mrak of his former colleague. Business possibilities related to the science and technology involved in feeding soldiers continue to this day.

A sampling of what's coming up next from the House of GI Joe follows. These vignettes describe projects ongoing in 2007, the year in which we looked closely at the Combat Feeding Program's activities, and are most of the important ones of the first decade of the twenty-first century. They fall into categories as diverse as shipping, storage, household appliances, personal devices, food safety, and dietary supplements, and are organized roughly by physical size from smallest to largest.

Pathogen Biosensors

Biosensors, bits of cells harnessed to electrical signal transmitters, are tiny alarms or measuring devices. They turn diagnoses that once took weeks of costly laboratory analysis with specialized equipment and trained personnel into tests that can be performed for pennies, on-site, in minutes, and by anyone. Two of these, the blood glucose monitor and the home pregnancy test, have been used for many years, but the military didn't get interested in biosensors until the 1980s, when the confluence of enzyme immobilization techniques, cloning, and genetic engineering gave our enemies the potential to mass-produce biological weapons.

The United States, constrained by the Geneva Protocol, and then by President Nixon's signing of the Biological Weapons Convention in 1972, could not retaliate in kind. But we could protect ourselves by figuring out how to detect accidental or weaponized pathogens. To provide "better defense against the threat of chemical and biological warfare," the army's Edgewood Chemical Biological Center organized the very first conferences on biosensors, one in 1985 that was attended by a scant two and a half dozen people, primarily army contractors, and another in 1988, which attracted a larger and more diverse audience, including many academics and industry members. By the early years of the twenty-first century, the private sector, seeing the potential in a technology that had applications in medicine, pharmaceuticals, food, and the environment, had taken up the baton. A journal on biosensors was founded, a yearly conference was held, and the global market was calculated in ever-increasing billions instead of millions.

However, the military still didn't have its pathogen detectors, which it now planned to use to test the military food supply in addition to identifying bioterrorism agents. It continued to fund their development during the 2000s through various basic and applied research contracts. One of those was as a small part of a $3.2 billion advanced electronics contract—mostly for air defense technology, air traffic control, and communications systems—between Hanscom Air Force Base's Electronic Systems Center and MIT's Lincoln Laboratory, from which, finally, came a rapid pathogen detection system called CANARY (patent application PCT/US2006/045691). Microchips are coated with arrays of white blood cells genetically modified to include a luminescent protein from fish; when a pathogen is detected, they light up, emitting photons. That system is now used in numerous commercial products, including the food pathogen detectors BioFlash-AF and Zephyr made by Maryland-based PathSensors. Another was a partnership with Michigan State University on a Department of Homeland Security contract, which developed nanofibers that could both capture pathogens and convey information about them to a reader. The result of this was a Michigan State University patent (patent application US 12/715,929) that was then licensed by nanoRETE, a start-up founded by the study's lead researcher (and patent holder). One of their first contracts was an air force Small Business Innovation Research (SBIR) award to apply their novel technology to tuberculosis detection; food pathogens are sure to follow.

Performance-Enhancing Ingredients and Novel Delivery Systems

Who doesn't have an acquaintance who swears by ginkgo biloba for his recent-onset senior moments, attributes her ability to refuse seconds of white chocolate raspberry cheesecake to green tea extract, or—seemingly paradoxically—downs gallons of saw palmetto tea at dinner to minimize his nocturnal perambulations? The military came late to the dietary supplement party, but when it joined, it joined with a vengeance. After the Dietary Supplement Health and Education Act of 1994 was passed, which stated that "the Federal Government should not take any actions to impose unreasonable regulatory barriers limiting or slowing the flow of safe products,"[5] the industry ballooned, growing from $4 billion in annual sales to $28 billion in 2010. The Combat Feeding Program, in partnership with the U.S. Army Research Institute of Environmental Medicine, which works on soldier nutrition, caught the fever. "The intent of the project is to take a look at naturally occurring food components that enhance cognitive or physical requirements on the battlefield," says Gerry Darsch, the Combat Feeding Directorate's former head. Since the early 2000s, a special team, the Performance Enhancement and Food Safety Team (PEFST), has conducted, commissioned, or been involved with numerous studies that identify bioactive substances, correlate their intake with a physical or cognitive change, attempt to elucidate their mechanism of action, set dose parameters, discover the best delivery routes, determine shelf stability, and taste-test them with civilians and soldiers. The result is a whole new set of rations, ones that not only satisfy hunger, but are doused with extracts and additives intended to improve performance.

The first round of ration supplements was developed over the period from 2000 through 2005 by the Natick food and environmental medicine departments and the Pennington Biomedical Research Center in Baton Rouge, Louisiana, which has received more than $40 million in Congressional Special Interest funding to work with different army centers since 1988. Their first projects focused on fatigue fighters, which they originally thought to deliver via transdermal patch, an idea that was quickly discarded when the team realized the molecules they wanted to transmit—proteins, carbohydrates, and fats—were too large to pass through skin. Efforts were shifted to buccal absorption through the cheek wall, which was achieved by holding a lozenge or gel in the mouth or by chewing gum, a chew, or a bar. A gel was developed composed of glucose, maltodextrin (a complex carbohydrate that digests more slowly), and a tiny bit of fat and protein that had a biphasic effect on blood sugar— a spike and then a rebound—making its impact last longer than that of commercially available products. The Natick Center also developed a maltodextrin-fortified applesauce, Zapplesauce, and a powdered energy drink, ERGO. In addition to carbohydrate loading, the PEFST group experimented with good old caffeine, which is considered critical in the military because they are often in "situations in which extended alertness is paramount" and "caffeine reverses sleep-deprivation induced degradation in cognitive performance."[6] The team found that buccal absorption was the quickest and most efficient way to get the psychoactive drug into the bloodstream, so they added it to chewing gum—it's now a standard part of the ration—and to the dense HooAH! energy bar, which was developed in a Cooperative Research and Development Agreement (CRADA) with the candy maker Mars in the early 2000s.

Between 2005 and the present, Natick extended its dietary supplement research to protein encapsulation, probiotics, amino acids, and phytonutrients. In 2007 it began adding encapsulated protein to the First Strike bar; this technique preserves flavor and prevents discoloration. It has continued to work on shelf stability for probiotics—including the construction of the first-ever "simulated digestion model" to estimate their absorption by the gut—and amino acids, and has been developing nanoscale carriers for micronutrients to add to ration components. Once fielded, this should be an important addition to the soldier's arsenal against food-borne illnesses; 76 percent of troops have at least one episode of diarrhea when deployed abroad. But what may have the most lasting impact on the consumer market is its phytonutrient research—although not in the way you might expect.

Plant flavonoids have received a lot of attention in the last couple of decades and have spawned a multimillion-dollar industry that sells the compounds in capsules and tablets. The Natick Center was curious—but cautious. As they observe, "There are many products on the market purported to have physiological benefits that may be of interest to the military. However, these products are typically classified as dietary supplements with little or no supporting research published in peer-reviewed journals."[7] Found in many fruits and vegetables and some grains, quercetin, the most common of these flavonoids, was touted as a way to increase energy. In 2006, with the assistance of the Rutgers University Ernest Mario School of Pharmacy in New Jersey, Natick began to test the compound's ability to delay onset of muscle fatigue and reduce muscle recovery time. "The results of clinical studies were intriguing, to say the least," says Darsch. "However, the consistency of the clinical studies seemed to be lacking.... So we brought the best scientists who'd been studying the effects of quercetin to Natick, [from] the American Institute of Biological Sciences. Some people felt it had ability to enhance mitochondrial biogenesis [growth of new mitochondria] within the cells. Mitochondria are like little engines in the body, an energy generator. We saw all sorts of data, some of it compelling, some of it not so compelling. As a result of bringing all of these world-class scientists together, we were able to have everybody present their respective information, and at the end of the day, it appeared that the effect of quercetin was individually specific." The Natick group added quercetin to a chew, the First Strike bar, and Tang in a follow-up study. Their results confirmed the findings of the conference: quercetin had a positive effect on some subjects, but variations in the bioavailability of the compound in the different food media, overall absorption, and enhancement effects were too great to be a reliable source of fatigue relief. The army discontinued the project.

Today, the army's fortification program largely relies on the old standbys: vitamins, minerals, carbohydrates, proteins, and caffeine. But it uses these liberally; in fact, in ration lines such as the First Strike, at least half the items have been fortified. Take Menu 1. Unadulterated—supplement-wise—are the shelf-stable pocket sandwiches, filled French toast, pretzel sticks, peanut butter dessert bar, sweet BBQ beef snack, and teriyaki beef snack. Pumped up are the jalapeño cheese spread (fortified with vitamins A, B_1, B_6, and D, and calcium), wheat snack bread (added calcium), chocolate Mini First Strike bar (just about everything), Cinnamon Zapplesauce (extra carbohydrates), nut and fruit mix (extra vitamin C), carbohydrate-fortified beverage, chocolate protein drink, cinnamon-flavored caffeinated gum, and sugar-free beverage (extra vitamin C).

Natick's caution when it comes to supplements is a good thing. With a mandate to use only peer-reviewed research, their investigations tend to be slow and careful. In the case of quercetin, which has an almost fanatical following in the supplement market, the Natick Center assessed its effect on the body, determined the most efficient medium for its delivery, and worked to understand its mode of action before ultimately deciding that the hype was unwarranted. In holding dietary supplements to a higher standard than those mandated by the FDA, they provide a public service. The world of over-the-counter "natural" medicine can be dangerous. High consumption of certain dietary supplements has been linked to severe illness and even death. Green tea extract can cause liver disease, and geranium extract, a stimulant, may have been the factor in the death of two soldiers in 2012 (a possibility that caused DOD to investigate it and ban its sale in base outlets). Fifty-three percent of soldiers use dietary supplements (a higher rate than for civilians), which gives the army a good reason to research these substances carefully and publicize the results. In response to the base deaths, the military launched a safety campaign that, among other things, gives soldiers access to a database where they can look up safety studies and adverse event reports on fifty-three thousand items. It would be great if this were open to the public. But meanwhile, the safest thing would be to follow Natick's example, and stick with the tried-and-true. Coffee run!

Extending the Shelf Life of FF&V (Fresh Fruits and Vegetables)

Even for modern warfighters, whose family dinners, like those of most Americans, were far more likely to have come from hastily heated bags and boxes or takeout than fresh ingredients cooked from scratch, an apple, a banana, a tomato, or a cucumber is a taste of paradise after long months on the battlefield. "Fresh fruits and vegetables are a morale enhancer, particularly for warfighters at forward operating bases who just don't get an option to eat anything resembling them," says Gerry Darsch. For this reason, the Defense Department pays billions of dollars through its prime vendor contracts to ensure a steady supply of fresh foods and staples. It costs so much not only because of the difficulty in transporting these items from third countries through war-torn nations to bases and camps, but also because the prolonged journey means more deterioration and spoilage, often rendering the product unusable.

Fresh fruits and vegetables are the most delicate of foodstuffs: easily bruised, they begin to decline the moment they are picked and respire, along with water vapor and carbon dioxide, the "death hormone." "Ethylene is a chemical compound that is emitted from fruits and vegetables that accelerates the ripening process. If you control it, it's a great thing. However, if you have a mixed load of FF&V, it can become your worst nightmare," explains Darsch. One of the goals of the Natick Center in the latter part of the first decade of the twenty-first century was to figure out a way to extend the shelf life of these perishables.

Unlike commercial produce vendors, the military usually ships an assortment of produce to serve in mess halls. Different fruits and vegetables have very different rates of ethylene production, so heavy respirers can hasten the spoilage of container mates. For example, the climacteric fruits, such as apples and bananas, that ripen after harvest are prolific ester factories—one part per million can condemn to the compost heap a whole shipment of lettuce in a single day. Until recently, ethylene levels were kept in check by using special filters for air purifiers in cold rooms, sachets and blankets placed by hand in boxes or chambers, and clay-based sorbents that work like kitty litter to remove gases. All of these methods are expensive and logistically difficult.

To find a way to reduce the presence of ethylene, Natick took its time-honored gladiator approach: it built up a couple of rivals, had them come up with a prototype, and then let them duel for the prize. It awarded two SBIR contracts, one to MicroEnergy Technologies, Inc., in Oregon and the other to Primaira in Massachusetts. Ultimately, MicroEnergy's solution, which combined electrocatalysis with an electrochemical sensor was "effective, but from a logistics perspective, that application, to be at its finest, in terms of return on investment, really had to be done right in the field where the fruits and vegetables were harvested," says Darsch. Primaira, on the other hand, focused their efforts on the creation of a small ultraviolet ozone device—with three hundred times more ozone than other machines—for cold rooms and containers that would break down any ethylene encountered to water and carbon dioxide. The apparatus was cheap, easy to use, required minimal power, and created no dangerous waste products: an investor's dream. "The UV light further acts to sanitize the air in the container by inactivating microbes, spores, and fungus," notes the army's write-up of the project.

From the outset, the Natick Center knew its ethylene zapper, which offers a seven-day extension over traditional methods, would have a market in commercial warehousing, transport, and retailer storage of produce. "We feel very confident that it's going to add considerable value not only to the warfighter but to the commercial logistics chain whose job it is to move things across the country. So we're kind of excited about that," says Darsch. It didn't take long. In early 2014 Maersk Container Industry, a specialty manufacturer of refrigerated containers, announced a partnership with Primaira to install the device, dubbed Bluezone, in their products. One of their first targets will be the $14 billion global fresh-cut flower business. Ninety percent of the intercontinental flower trade is shipped by air, which greatly increases the cost of production; if this could be done in reefers, it would revolutionize the industry. "We are still working on the final design, but we are convinced that the Blue-zone and Star Cool combination represents economic and environmental upsides so far unseen in container transportation," says Soren Leth Johannsen, chief commercial officer of Maersk Container Industry in *Food Logistics* magazine.

Another important issue with the salads and fresh fruits served in mess halls is the potential presence of pathogenic bacteria. The produce provided by DOD's prime contractors to foreign bases often comes from neighboring countries—in which livestock, crops, and facilities-deprived laborers may intermingle. By 2005, the Natick Center began to research the possibility of inoculating fresh plant products with viruses that infect *Salmonella, E. coli* O157:H7 (the potentially deadly strain), and *Shigella*, all mesophiles that thrive in human intestines and are spread via fecal contamination. They granted multiple SBIR and Small Business Technology Transfer awards to Intralytix, a biotech company based in Baltimore, Maryland, that specializes in genetic engineering of bacteriophages (viruses that infect specific bacteria). The company developed separate products for each bacterial menace; they could be sprayed singly or in a mixed cocktail on suspect fresh foods.

By 2009 Intralytix was into its third cycle of awards from the army; the last round was intended to help the company commercialize its *E. coli* product—paying for everything from business plans and investment planning to "facilitation of meetings with potential private or government customers."[8] In 2011 the company's *E. coli* spray was approved by both the FDA and the USDA for use "on red meat parts and trim intended to be ground."[9] The chief scientist of Intralytix, Alexander Sulakvelidze, explained in an e-mail, "Even though no patents resulted from the work funded by Natick, their support was instrumental in getting critical efficacy data, securing regulatory approvals for EcoShield, and helping with its large scale-up production—all vital components for the commercialization." A few months after it received regulatory approval, the company entered into a multiproject agreement with Procter & Gamble. In 2013, its SalmoFresh anti-*Salmonella* spray was given GRAS status by the FDA. This is just the beginning. Given increasing consumer concerns about food-borne illnesses—one of the impetuses behind the Food Safety Modernization Act—the demand for products such as those developed by Intralytix should only increase.

Individual Beverage Chillers

You're hiking through the sand, lugging 130 pounds of gear, sweltering in the midday sun. You take a refreshing sip from the hose of your CamelBak hydration system—and gag. Just try replacing the up to two liters of fluids lost per hour in desert climates when all you have to drink is hot disinfectant-flavored water. Heat-related dehydration is responsible for between fifteen hundred and two thousand cases of heat exhaustion, heat stroke, and death per year in the services; untold illnesses; and a generalized decline in warrior physical and cognitive performance. The simple fix is a nice, cool drink.

To encourage soldiers to take more fluids while in action, the military decided in 2004 to chill individual water packs; it entered into the first of two SBIR contracts with Creare, an engineering company in Hanover, New Hampshire (from FY 2000 through FY 2012, the firm earned a cool $159 million in DOD contracts). The engineers came up with a small battery-operated refrigeration system that could be attached to an existing water system, cooling just the reservoir before the liquid goes into the drinking hose. Around the same time, Natick entered into a CRADA with the military supplier BCB International to develop a version of the chiller that didn't need a power source at all; instead, it worked through a series of twelve evaporating wicks. Neither design was perfect: the water could only be cooled by 35°F–40°F, bringing the temperature down to merely tepid, but at least it was drinkable. In 2010 both models were field-tested by marines in the Mojave Desert. BCB's invention, the Chilly, left the Creare device in the dust, winning the approbation of more than two-thirds of the evaluators; now trademarked, it has already made inroads in the commercial market through sales to the next generation of adopters—skiers, cyclists, hikers, and long-distance runners.

Solar-Powered Refrigerated Containers

The extended twenty-first-century American sojourn in the Middle East could well be called the containerized war. These corrugated steel boxes, the inspiration of a North Carolina trucker who was vexed by the amount of time it took to load and unload boxes by hand, made seamless the transfer of goods from truck to train to ship. By the end of the twentieth century, the classic "disruptive technology" had achieved world domination, and the numbers of containers only continue to grow—in 2012 there were 32.9 million. In Afghanistan and Iraq, the U.S. Armed Forces use containers for just about everything: they serve as maintenance shops, dog kennels, laundry units, weapons rooms, and clean rooms, and are the way all goods are shipped, stored, and, of course, refrigerated. Because of their cooling machinery, refrigerated containers, called reefers, cost as much as ten times more than a regular container (up to $30,000) and are expensive to run, as they must continually be fed electricity to maintain the cold chain. The army has solved this problem on its bases by using portable generators that run on JP-8 (a less combustible jet propellant that fuels all army equipment), but over the course of a year, each refrigerated container can suck up seven thousand to nine thousand gallons of fuel.

Thus, there was nothing particularly environmentalist about the army's embrace of sustainable energy. The wars in Iraq and Afghanistan, fought in and over the land of petroleum, have had the most expensive fuel costs ever, in both financial and human terms. Seventy percent of the vehicles in convoys were fuel trucks; each burned seven gallons of fuel for every one it delivered to a base; en route they were at constant risk for attack and required protection in the form of air cover, tracking devices, and video monitoring, which upped the costs even more. The solution? To hell with the supply chain. An Iraq War commander, Commanding General Richard Zilmer, chief of Multi-National Force West, sent a memo to the Pentagon in 2006, urging it to find sustainable sources of energy: "By reducing the need for [petroleum-based fuels] at our outlying bases, we can decrease the frequency of logistics convoys on the road, thereby reducing the danger to our Marines, soldiers, and sailors."[10]

The Natick Center's solar-powered refrigerated container was in the right place at the right time. Two different companies had been contracted to develop the technology and equipment. Starting in FY 2004, an SBIR award was given to Mainstream Engineering in Florida, a refrigeration and energy engineering company and longtime DOD contractor, to investigate the feasibility of mounting photovoltaic cells on container roofs, to demo a new cooling and energy storage system, and then to build a single prototype solar-powered reefer. SunDanzer, a tiny company specializing in solar-powered refrigeration in Arizona and started by a former NASA contractor (DOD quickly became its biggest and practically only client), was awarded an SBIR contract in FY 2006 for the same purpose and another one to create a $3,500-per-unit passive-cooling retrofit for the containers used to store semiperishables (U.S. Patent 6,253,563, originally assigned to NASA). (There was also a 2007–10 contracting blip, a hallowed tradition known as the congressional plus-up—the Pentagon's own private term for the numerous earmarks its friends in the House and Senate tack onto its budget—that resulted in an almost million-dollar Broad Agency Agreement with a third company, Advanced Technology Materials Incorporated in Connecticut, to develop a solar-powered adsorption refrigerator in a Quadcon, an army-developed minicontainer a quarter of the size of a regular one. Despite a scintillating ninety-two-page report, its prototype failed to meet minimum performance standards, and the project was scrapped.) In 2010 SunDanzer was chosen to finalize development of the integrated solar-powered container system, and the equipment is scheduled to be incorporated into field kitchens in FY 2016. (Mainstream Engineering, the first contractor, was also graced with a $40 million contract for the production of new insulated Tricon containers equipped with the company's new high-performance/energy-efficient refrigeration unit, but without the solar energy component.) If the technology gains traction in the commercial marketplace, there are more than two million reefers circling the globe just waiting to be liberated from the power grid.

Waste-to-Energy Converters

Just like you, the army has bills. And just like you, the bills it hates the most are the humongous ones it has for fuel and garbage disposal (done the traditional way by burning or landfill). Each soldier generates approximately eight pounds of solid waste daily, 80 percent of which is food related. Was there a way to efficiently and economically turn their garbage into a power source to run the many generators—twenty-seven per 550 soldiers—that dot each base?

The idea, of course, is nothing new. People have been burning garbage since ancient times and, starting in the late 1800s, have done so on a large scale in machines designed for the purpose. Engineers quickly figured out how to capture some of the heat energy by turning it into steam, which could then be used to drive a turbine, but energy recovery didn't really take off until after the oil price shocks and the "give a hoot, don't pollute" activism of the 1970s. There are now about 450 waste-to-energy incinerators in Europe and 100 in the United States. But while torching trash reduced the burden of waste disposal for municipalities, it still generated toxic compounds, carbon dioxide, carbon monoxide, and a great deal of ash. Even worse, it's a really lousy way to harvest the energy locked within.

Several promising new energy recovery technologies had appeared by the 1990s; they were based, as is combustion, on the effect of high heat and air on organic material—sort of deconstructing fire into its by-products (gas, oil, char). Combustion, the old standby, occurs at 800°F–1,200°F in an oxygen-rich environment. This bathes every component of the fuel in oxygen, producing a whole family of little "-ides"—carbon dioxide, sulfur dioxide, nitrogen oxide—and water, none of which can be burned, so any energy transfer has to happen through water vapor.

Combustion's efficiency is a flaccid 15–25 percent. Gasification also happens at 800°F–1200°F, but in an oxygen-limited environment that forces more of the components of the fuel to become a flammable gas called syngas; it burns with an efficiency of 30–40 percent. Pyrolysis occurs at lower temperatures, 300°F–600°F, but in the complete absence of oxygen, so the organic material is rendered into a flammable bio-oil. When ignited, it burns with an efficiency of 35–45 percent, but it's highly corrosive, so isn't suitable for engines. A final option, one not dependent on the application of heat to biomass, is supercritical water depolymerization. Intimidating polysyllabic name notwithstanding, it simply means subjecting water to both high temperatures and high pressure. This pushes the water molecules close as if they were in a liquid, but because they are excited by all the thermal energy, there is much less hydrogen bonding. The excess of available hydrogen turns supercritical water into both a strong acid and a strong base, so it can dissolve just about anything, even the plastics and paperboard that riddle our rubbish.

Finding a workable waste-to-energy conversion model was an army-wide goal for the twenty-first century; multiple research agencies, including the Defense Advanced Research Projects Agency (DARPA), the U.S. Army Research Laboratory, and Natick, took up the challenge. Eight prototypes were eventually developed; in 2007 four of these, the ones most suitable for use in field kitchens, were under consideration by Natick. The first was a DARPA project with General Atomics, a major California defense contractor—they were awarded $2.4 billion in government contracts in 2012 alone—to develop a converter using supercritical water. The other three were Natick initiatives funded through the SBIR program: two gasifiers—one from Community Power Corporation (CPC) in Colorado and one from Infoscitex Corporation in Massachusetts—and a pyrolysis-based model built by Green Liquid & Gas Technologies in Florida. All four companies had presented prototypes, and the Combat Feeding Program selected two, CPC's gasifier and General Atomics' supercritical water depolymerization process, for further refinement and field testing. In 2010 the army asked CPC to produce its BioMax system (U.S. Patent 7,909,899), which uses air to push the gases downward for collection instead of up, thereby reducing emissions, for further modifications and yet another field test. At the same time, they asked Infoscitex Corporation to develop on its own a prototype using the same process, combined with its initial innovation of using shredded (rather than pelletized) waste, which is cleaner, faster, and more efficient (U.S. patent application PCT/US2011/001972). While neither model has been fielded yet, both companies have entered the commercial market as an environmentally friendly alternative to incineration or trucking waste to landfills.

★ ★ ★

THE ARMY CALLS THIS "HIGH RISK, HIGH PAYOFF" research and development. While each of these inventions has the potential for spin-offs in the broader realm of resource conservation, bioengineering, nanotechnology, food preservation, and human health, and perhaps to impact the consumer food market in the years and decades to come, there are no guarantees. Some approaches and companies will succeed; others will not. But for the venture capitalist who is willing to invest at the very edges of science and technology, the opportunities await.

Chapter 14

DO WE REALLY WANT OUR CHILDREN EATING LIKE SPECIAL OPS?

The wars of tomorrow will be lonely places. Whether nuclear, conventional, or unconventional, they will often rely on tactics developed for small units of special operations forces: reconnaissance and surveillance; partner support and training; low-intensity fighting, infiltration, prevention, and response to terrorist acts; and destruction of high-value targets, human or otherwise. In this fluid and dynamic battle environment, large garrisons, with their complicated and expensive infrastructure, will be burdensome to set up, supply, and operate. Logistics support will be shifted to small forward operating bases, which can be installed from containers in a matter of two weeks anywhere in the world, as well as to the even more minimally equipped outposts the military calls "austere."

Army camps are being downsized for strategic and cost reasons and because the individual soldier system—everything a warrior needs to sustain her except for weapons—will soon be exponentially more powerful. During the past decade, the Natick Center has been working with MIT and industrial partners, including its old chums Raytheon and DuPont, on body armor built of nanomaterials that give warriors unprecedented capabilities and self-sufficiency: networked communications;

surveillance and geographic coordination; detection and neutralization of biological and chemical contaminants; temperature and hydration control; and constant physiological monitoring with as-needed administration of medical treatment and performance boosters. At the same time, the warfighter will be frighteningly dependent—on technology, on a power source (this wrinkle hasn't quite yet been solved), and on the communications network. He will be given superhuman powers—to see at night, to change appearance (perhaps even to be invisible), and to walk through a hail of bullets, yet have reduced agency in making decisions on the battlefield and even about his own body.

There's not a lot of room for a hot, sit-down meal for eight, ten, or twelve in this scenario.

But there will be an even greater need for a diverse range of rugged, shelf-stable foods that can be stored anywhere and eaten out of hand. And this suits the military just fine. Because as it turns out, despite the higher processing and packaging costs, combat rations are the army's most cost-effective feeding method. No need to set up battlefield kitchens with all their energy-hungry machines. No need to ship perishables or arrange for dodgy third-country purveyors. No veterinary inspectors breathing down your neck. No refrigerated containers. No surly cooks. No kitchen waste to dispose of, pots to scrub, equipment to scrape, and mess halls to maintain. Just tear, eat, and toss. And then run your fan or charge your phone or play Xbox on the energy the waste-to-energy converter provides from your trash.

In fact, the army is close to scrapping the meal concept entirely. "We're looking at, is three meals a day really the way we want to feed warfighters?" says Gerry Darsch, the former director of the Combat Feeding Directorate. "Do we want to make it more of a grazing event, rather than a specific 'this is a breakfast, this is a lunch, this is a dinner.' . . . We're looking at convenience, eating on the move, yet still providing that nutritional core that warfighters need."

Which means that Natick will continue to do what it's been doing, only more so.

★ ★ ★

WRITING THIS BOOK CHANGED ME. I'm no longer a home-cooking fanatic. Nor do I believe that industrial food—and by extension, those involved in its design and production—is inherently evil. I'm also way more comfortable talking about science and engineering than I ever believed possible. And at the supermarket, I see ghosts everywhere, watered-down combat rations filling shelves, refrigerator cases, and bins.

My epiphany came a year into the project, during the first ever visit of my Cuban mother-in-law, who, practically on arrival, took over my kitchen. She did things Latin American style—rising at dawn, preparing everything from fresh ingredients, making huge quantities. On the penultimate day of her stay, I asked my husband what one childhood dish did he want me to learn so that I could reincarnate the taste of his long-ago home. To my surprise—whither the Cuban soul food, *frijoles negros*?—he wanted a citrus, garlic, and oregano–marinated chicken. His mother wrote out a list of ingredients, and he set out for Whole Foods, returning with jars of spices, bottles of olive oil, kosher salt, perfectly globular onions, garlic, bags of lemons and limes, and two rosy chickens fed only organic grain and raised free-range.

At the appointed time, I stepped into the kitchen, tied on an apron, whipped out my reporter's notebook, and stood at attention. Melba had unwrapped the chickens and placed them on the cutting board, backsides up like two naughty children. She slid a kitchen knife out of the block. "First you cut the legs off, *así*," she said, easing the blade around the bone. She spent twenty minutes carefully dismembering the carcasses and placing pieces one by one in a glass baking dish as I scribbled furiously. She then filled a plastic bag with giblets, backbones, and wings. "What are you doing?" I asked. "Oh"—as she tossed the bag into the freezer—"We don't need these. Maybe you can use them later?" I made a large X through the page of handwritten directions. "Two packages of drumsticks and breasts," I wrote. A year or two ago, I would have followed her instructions to a T, convinced that doing it myself somehow made it better. It was the moment when I understood I'd gone to the other side.

Of course, a year or two earlier, I hadn't had a mammoth project and a scary deadline. Since I began *Combat-Ready Kitchen,* there have been very few moments when I wasn't working on it, if not at my computer, then in my head. In the past, the hour or so in the kitchen preparing a sit-down meal for six had relaxed me. Now I resented it. As the owner of a public health communications agency, I had always had a fairly good work-life balance (if zero recreation): I worked from a home office, I spent time with my kids, I cooked. Now my life had no balance. I researched and I wrote, and when I wasn't researching and writing, I was worrying about researching and writing. This frame of mind did not lend itself well to the unhurried ritual of chop-sauté-serve.

My new mantra became "How quickly can I open a bunch of boxes and bags and get something on the table?" Gone were my braised lamb, my *sancocho,* my squash soups with tiny, garlicky meatballs. In with spaghetti, jarred sauce, and pregrated cheese. Vegetarian burritos with canned refried beans and some shredded cabbage and carrots. Frozen pizza (a lot of frozen pizza). I suddenly had more sympathy for the typical working mother's dilemma, and more tolerance for take-out and ready-to-serve food. We were tired. We were overstretched. Something had to give, and that something was dinner. And you know what? Good riddance.

Cooking, like music before it, is a dying art, moving from the precincts of the private and personal—our great-grandparents sang and played instruments—to the realm of the public and commercial. Now when I "cook" for my family, chances are that at least half, if not all, of the components and ingredients have been processed in some way. Behind my takeout stands an officer corps of master chefs, an army of food-service workers, and a few mammoth suppliers that have cracked the prepared food nut. Behind my ready-to-eat meals stands a small city's worth of food scientists and engineers and the vast, hyperefficient machinery of American agribusiness, food processors, packers, shippers, and retailers. And behind them, like a shadowy puppeteer, stands the one entity to which having inexpensive, portable, long-shelf-life, easy-to-prepare or ready-to-eat food is vitally important, at times existentially so: the U.S. Army.

In significant part because of military influence, food science has made breathtaking strides during the twentieth century and now the twenty-first. Understanding what makes food taste good—as well as be safe and be able to be stored without deterioration—is no longer an art, know-how accumulated through painstaking observation and assiduously passed down through the generations, but a science. That is to say, a body of knowledge based on observable facts, precise principles, and repeatable experiments. This has turbocharged food preparation. We may have been making bread, cheese, ham, and jam since almost the dawn of time, but understanding the mechanisms at work, and being able to predict and control them, is what makes industrial food possible as well as sparking the invention of thousands of new edibles. The 1956 promise made by George Larrick, then commissioner of the FDA, the agency that oversees new food-processing technology, has been fulfilled: "I can predict that the housewife of the future will practice the art of cooking only occasionally as a hobby."[1]

That describes me perfectly, and is the reason for which to all these actors I give—qualified—thanks. On the one hand, they've offered me unprecedented freedom: freedom from drudgery, freedom to do more of what I like and want—whether that's watching hours of reality TV or saving the lives of children in poor countries by distributing oral rehydration therapy.* In the past, I'd chosen to cook the old-fashioned way. But creatively, writing a book was way more fulfilling than even my most inspired meals—assemblages of ingredients that pleased the eye, tickled the palate, and soothed, if only momentarily, the soul. So now I was making another choice. What's important is not to condemn one another

---

* Every year almost a million children die from diarrhea, deaths that could be easily prevented with inexpensive oral rehydration salts. See *Ending Preventable Child Deaths from Pneumonia and Diarrhoea by 2025: The Integrated Global Action Plan for the Prevention and Control of Pneumonia and Diarrhoea (GAPPD)* (United Nations Children Fund, World Health Organization, 2013).

for our decisions on how to eat, but to recognize how incredibly lucky and privileged we twenty-first-century women—yes, I'm going to gender this—are, in that we have a choice.

On the other hand, many, but not all, industrial foods are unhealthy, high in sugar, salt, and fat and low in fiber, vitamins, and minerals. Just as bad—or even worse—to achieve stability and long shelf life, they contain numerous additives, from chemical preservatives and antimicrobials to gums and fillers. Many of these "ingredients" have never before been eaten or eaten in such quantities, and we know little or nothing about their long-term effects. But despite this and perhaps contrary to what you might expect, I am now cautiously optimistic about the possibility—and the slowly growing reality—that we can have food that is both convenient and good for us. If other values besides those that are militarily necessary were at the forefront of government, academic, and industry food research, we might be able to add yet another choice to the menu, one that caters to the concerns of women, and increasingly men, who want to put delicious, wholesome dinners on the table quickly and affordably. (The army, to its credit, wants this, too, and, in fact, has spearheaded next-generation processing techniques that, if they prove to be comparable in safety to fresh food, may help us do just that.)

★ ★ ★

IN LOCKSTEP WITH THE MILITARY'S PROGRESSION from World War II's K rations to the War on Terror's First Strike Rations, with its cornucopia of sandwiches, wraps, pizza, energy bars, savory snacks, and candy, the industrial food system has increasingly supplied us with items that can be eaten as is or require only heating. The Defense Department's goal is to "provide the best possible rations to soldiers," a task that it foresees will include "continued reduction in weight, volume and equipment energy consumption, improvements in phytonutrient validation and delivery, shelf life optimization, and the ongoing need to meet the changing needs of the military as its mission continues to adapt to changing conflicts."[2] That's as it should be. But we consumers don't have to accept a food system coupled to military feeding.

The first step is to realize that the U.S. Army, by being almost the sole investor in the big issues in food science and groundbreaking technology and then by purposefully seeding the results in industry—both to maintain the industrial base during peacetime and to lower the cost and improve related products—to a large degree controls the general direction of the American diet. This book should help you see that. But even after my two and a half years of research, it only scratches the surface; a thorough treatise on the topic would require dozens of volumes and a cadre of academics eager to devote their careers to it.

The second step is to pry the decision-making process that guides the Combat Feeding Program from exclusively military hands and bring in actors who can consider the impact of the kinds of science and technology it invests in on the rest of us. For many years, the Natick Center's science program was overseen by a committee organized by the National Academy of Sciences–National Research Council and composed not only of Natick Center staff but of outside scientists and industry members. In the 1980s Natick reassigned that function solely to its military "customers." It's time to open up that decision-making process again, not only to academics and food businesses but to all those who feel its secondary effects—farmers, nutritionists, public health experts, and consumers.

A third step is to do more studies on the possible long-term effects on human health of these new techniques and products. It's great that high-pressure processing kills bacteria, but what about other physicochemical changes brought about by applying this immense force to food molecules? The studies related to human health are just starting to appear. We may have better vitamin retention, but what about the harmful effects of increased lipid oxidation—leading to the formation of those notorious troublemakers, the free radicals? And while we're at it, what about the two-, ten-, or twenty-year impact of regular ingestion of an infinitesimally small amount of the "generally recognized as safe" ingredients on the label or "reaction products" such as the acrylamides in the crackers your child nibbles all day? And, yes, cancer is terrible, but how about trying to understand how processing techniques and processed foods impact more systemic diseases and conditions, which, perhaps because they are more difficult to test for in the lab, have gotten short shrift?

Which brings us to a certain creaky regulatory agency long due for an overhaul: the FDA.* When its predecessor bureau in the USDA was given powers to protect consumers in 1906, and through 1938, when these were greatly expanded, the big issues in food were deceptive labeling and adulteration (bad stuff that isn't supposed to be in there, like melamine-tainted Chinese milk). In the late 1950s, its mandate was extended to additives and colors, after which Congress declared exempt several hundred substances it considered to be generally recognized as safe (GRAS); by 2010 that list had grown to more than nine thousand items (an additional one thousand have been approved by the industry as GRAS without FDA review[3]). In 2011, after a decade punctuated by bacteria-related outbreaks, President Barack Obama signed into law the Food Safety Modernization Act, which strengthened the government's ability to monitor and detect food-borne illnesses.

But many of the FDA's scientific frameworks, regulatory approaches, and enforcement policies are still inadequate to protect the public from potential dangers in our food. The "harm" standard should be clearly defined and include low-level exposures over long periods, and how they may contribute to a whole range of diseases, not just the Big C, but allergies, autoimmune conditions, reproductive and endocrine issues, and, of course, public enemy number one: obesity and his pasty pals hypertension, heart disease, and diabetes. And to make informed choices about what we buy, we need a lot more information than an (incomplete) list of ingredients. The FDA should promote transparency about how industrial food is made and require companies to publish—if not on the label, then on their Web sites or on the FDA's—information about their products' processing technologies, temporary additives (that may disappear or leave only traces), new substances created in manufacturing, and migration of materials into food during processing and from packaging,

---

* The FDA categorically refused to be interviewed for this book.

as well as the possible health effects of the same. Finally, it must also require that same transparency of itself by creating public records of the regulatory process, even informal communications, and install vigilant external watchdogs over, or avoid altogether, collaborations that result in products that come under its own purview.

What would our food be like if the Natick Center didn't exist? If there wasn't an invisible—at least to the consumer and most industry members—force relentlessly driving consumer products toward the military ideal of cheap, imperishable, and easy to store and transport? The question is unanswerable, because, in many ways, the work done by the Natick Center is the skeleton of industrial food. "Every kind of processing that we now have, at one time or another Natick was very interested in and would have put resources into," sums up food scientist and editor Daryl Lund. Remove the scientific and technological backbone on which the giant conglomerates adhere the last little bit of eye-fooling, appetite-tricking razzle-dazzle and everything collapses.

There's a watered-down combat ration lurking in practically every bag, box, can, bottle, jar, and carton we buy. This food, originally designed for soldiers, is bad for our health and the health of our children—at least when consumed, as do warriors and most of the rest of us, day in, day out, year after year. We're participating in a massive public health experiment, one in which science and technology, at the beck of the military, have taken over our kitchens. What are the long-term effects of such a diet? We really don't know: we're the guinea pigs.

★ ★ ★

AS IT TURNED OUT, the only person in my house perfectly happy to eat things out of cans, pouches, tubs, and boxes was me: I'd be fine munching crudités with dip, huge Greek salads, and tuna fish sandwiches for the rest of my life. My husband and I met when I ran a newsmagazine and he was an editor, and we ate almost all our meals at the dozens of inexpensive restaurants that stud Quito's neighborhoods, from open-air *cevicherías* to homey *comedores* (diners). It wasn't until two years later, after we'd married and returned to the United States, that he discovered my culinary talents, a matrimonial windfall that he enthusiastically accepted as his due. My children, on the other hand, grew up with me in the kitchen—literally; they sat across the cutout counter from me on stools. Although they may not be able to articulate it, the sight, sound, and smells that came as I turned to the four cardinal points of my perfect cook's circle—gas stove, sink, counter, refrigerator—must powerfully evoke home, safety, and maternal love.

Once I'd withdrawn from leisurely cooking and the sacred rite of the family dinner, everyone found a way to coax me to feed them. My husband, taking advantage of some spouse-approved tasks such as writing invoices, requested that I fix him a sandwich; my ham and cheese was, apparently, tastier than his. At night, my elderly mother would ask plaintively from the empty dining room table, "What do you want me to eat?" Implicit in this question was that I heat up some soup for her or set out a plate of cheese and crackers. And even though I'd inured them from an early age to sharp knives and dancing flames, my younger children requested pasta and quesadillas that they easily could have prepared themselves. I realized that what they sought wasn't my cooking, but the feeling that I was taking care of them. That I was their mother, wife, daughter. There are plenty of other ways to honor this connection, but cooking had always been one of mine. So as soon as this manuscript is shipped off to be printed, I'm heading back to the kitchen to simmer sustainably raised meats and organic vegetables in my 1920s cast-iron Dutch oven and frying pans—at least until the book comes out. And then who knows?

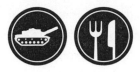

In 1987 we deployed to an unimproved airstrip in the middle of the Honduran jungle. Our mission wasn't very clear. It was in the middle of nowhere, no city or town anywhere close. I was E3, a lance corporal at the time. In the Marine Corps, E1s through E3s are always put on guard duty, so I was assigned to a post at a sandbag bunker improvised alongside the airstrip.

On my very first shift, out of the jungle came four or five little kids, maybe three to eight years old. I remember how frail and poor they were. None of the children had shoes, and all were filthy. They came out cautiously. They looked at us; we looked at them. We wanted to communicate with them, but they didn't speak English, and we didn't speak their native language. We couldn't let them get close because we were carrying live ammunition and loaded weapons. They went back into the jungle after that, but came back a little later. And this time they were a big group, maybe twenty kids. I still have the picture I took of them standing with the other guy on duty.

We had MREs that we'd been given to eat for lunch. We'd been told not to feed the indigenous children. The commander said, "You're really not helping them." But I had a hard time looking at those children knowing that they were in need. So I opened up my MRE, and I took a set of four square pieces of cracker inside a vacuum-sealed package. I motioned to the kids, holding it like I was going to fling it in the air. But they started to get a little crazy, so instead of doing that, I had one of the younger kids come closer and I gave it to him. And then he ran off from the group into the jungle. There was a bunch of them that followed. I emptied the whole MRE and the other marine's, too. Once the MREs were gone, the kids went back into the jungle. I was there at that location for about a month, and I did that often. I'm sure the other guys did, too, but nobody really talked about it because of the commander not wanting us to feed them.

When I got back to Camp Pendleton in the States, what I'd seen sunk into me. I had a newborn daughter, and I thought about the life I was fortunate enough to have, and the one my child was fortunate enough to have. I'd seen children I could tell were starving. Before then, I'd complained about the meals—that I didn't like them or they made me constipated. That experience humbled me and taught me to appreciate what I have in life. There are people out there that would do anything to get what you've got. I never looked at an MRE the same way after that.

—Sergeant Michael Eugene Kent Jr., United States Marine Corps, continental United States and Honduras, 1985–93

Acknowledgments

It can't have been easy for the Natick Center to have me as their unofficial biographer. On my first visit they were braced for the worst from "the bad girl of American food writing," a moniker I'd given myself in a moment of poor impulse control, and which they'd unearthed in an exhaustive Internet search, the results of which couldn't have been reassuring as to my intentions or methods. Nonetheless, they put their game face on. Represented by able public affairs officer David Accetta, the Combat Feeding Program hosted my visits, complied with my requests for interviews and materials, and even gave me referrals and suggestions, all with the utmost courtesy and alacrity. In the process, I developed a deep admiration for their corps of committed staff—civilian and military; scientific, technical, and administrative—who make the whole thing work, including their historically minded director, Stephen Moody. I was also privileged to be able to interview, solicit advice from, and have review the chapter on recent projects the indefatigable former director Gerry Darsch. Natick Center, I salute you!

Food scientists—and a few "regular" scientists—were a group indispensable to the making of this book and for whose knowledge, diligence, and generosity I gained an immense appreciation. Several read drafts of the science sections; to a one, they were swift, careful, and thorough, going back and forth with me for multiple rounds until the wording was perfect. Martin Cole, chief of the Australian Commonwealth Scientific and Industrial Research Organization's (CSIRO) Animal, Food, and Health Sciences division, despite being one of the world's busiest men, cheerfully made time for several interviews with me, answered questions by e-mail, and volunteered to review the lengthiest science piece in the book, on food microbiology. The paragraphs on light and heat and their effect on food deterioration benefited from New York University physicist Andrew MacFadyen's eagle eye. Dutch process-engineering professor Solke Bruin and German food engineer, peripatetic professor, and past president of the International Union of Food Science and Technology Walter Speiss offered invaluable feedback on the sections on freeze-drying, water activity, and intermediate-moisture foods. New Zealand meat scientist Mustafa Farouk both checked a time line of restructured meats and read the section on meat science. Dutch microbiology professor Nanne Nanninga shared with me his comprehensive understanding of yeast and his knowledge of the life of Van Leeuwenhoek. Food chemist and head of the CSIRO Food Science Research Program Mary Ann Augustin, as a generalist, and Purdue University carbohydrate chemist James Bemiller, as an expert, read through the section on bread staling and the application of polymer theory to same; renowned Irish dairy chemist and cheese expert Patrick Fox spotted me on the chapter that included processed cheese and cheese powder. Australian professor and consultant Gordon Robertson, one of the world's leading experts on food packaging, helped me explain polymer science in layman's terms without sacrificing accuracy in the underlying concepts and terms. Natural Resources Defense Council (NRDC) senior scientist Maricel Maffini and West Virginia University pharmaceutical science professor Vince Castranova read through the pages on phthalates and nanoparticles and gave feedback so that these reflected current science and health considerations. Investigative food scientist and consultant Kathryn Kotula made sure that my description of hurdle technology was faithful to the ideas espoused by Lothar Leistner, and Oregon State University food technologist Dan Farkas, in his inimitable lively manner, aided me in hammering out a description of high-pressure processing. NRDC chemical engineer and attorney Tom Neltner uncomplainingly interrupted his holiday break to improve my comprehension of the scope of the FDA's responsibilities and activities in regulating food additives and food-contact substances, as well as critiquing my recommendation about the same. Last but not least, food scientist and engineer and former editor of the *Journal of Food Science,* Daryl Lund, reviewed, added to, and approved the table of important twentieth- and twenty-first-century food science and technology developments I made as a roadmap before starting *Combat-Ready Kitchen.* Ladies and gentlemen, I was honored to be allowed a glimpse into the inner workings of your field and heartened to be treated with such kindness.

Long live librarians! The breed is now more important than ever to navigate the patchy quilt of online resources—some of which are open to all but poorly marked, and others of which are inaccessible to most unless you have an institutional affiliation. Several of these trusty individuals went beyond the call of duty in helping me with my research. Thanks to National Academy of Sciences archivist Janice Goldblum for the towering stack of documents she exhumed for me to peruse and for tolerating the cairns of Post-it-dotted files with which I littered the antechamber to her office. MIT Institute Archives and Special Collections reference associate Myles Crowley and the rest of the staff assembled an impressive showing of MIT–Quartermaster Corps projects and pulled boxes for me at the drop of a hat. University of California, Davis's Axel Borg, food science librarian extraordinaire, gave me the lay of the land in terms of the field's key publications and databases. Although we never spoke, Wayne Olson, reference librarian at the National Agricultural Library, compiled an extensive set of reports on and references to projects that were collaborations between the USDA and the army. And finally, although I follow a "first always, last never," rule in using it, I'm grateful to wikipedia.org for its mission of providing an unfettered entrance to the world's knowledge.

I had two constant companions in this journey; their specific contributions are too numerous to recount. Three cheers for my wonderful agent, Stephany Evans, who combines all the traits you'd most want in your advocate (or your mom, for that matter)—wisdom, warmth, and infallible good sense. I so appreciate your unflagging faith in me and my ideas. My editor, Emily Angell, miraculously found the perfect balance between giving me the creative leeway I needed to research, organize, and write, while questioning my sometimes questionable taste and pressing me to add countless details that enriched the stories. Equally miraculously, she remained pleasant, despite being on the receiving end of rather a lot of late-night authorial zingers in the manuscript's comments column. Kudos on your consummate professionalism! And one more shout-out: Maureen Clark, our relationship was brief and intense, but your meticulous copyediting immeasurably improved both the accuracy and the prose of *Combat-Ready Kitchen*. Hats off to you and the rest of the Current team, including senior production editor Bruce Giffords, art director Christopher Sergio, jacket designer Zoe Norvell, interior designer Daniel Lagin, and editorial assistant Kary Perez.

Notes

CHAPTER 2. AMERICAN FOOD SYSTEM, CENTRAL COMMAND, PART ONE

1. Valerie Bailey Grasso, *Department of Defense Food Procurement: Background and Status,* CRS Report No. RS22190 (Washington, DC: Congressional Research Service, Library of Congress, January 24, 2013).

CHAPTER 3. AMERICAN FOOD SYSTEM, CENTRAL COMMAND, PART TWO

1. House Committee on Armed Services, *Challenges to Doing Business with the Department of Defense: Findings of the Panel on Business Challenges in the Defense Industry* (Washington, DC, March 19, 2012), 48.
2. The defense industrial base is the "DOD, government, and the private sector worldwide industrial complex with the capabilities of performing research and development, design, production, delivery, and maintenance of military weapons systems, subsystems, components, or parts to meet military requirements," according to the Department of Homeland Security in *Principles of Emergency Management and Emergency Operations Centers (EOC)* edited by Michael J. Fagel (Boca Raton, FL: CRC Press, 2011). Although the researchers and manufacturers involved in developing and improving soldier food may not depend exclusively on the military for revenues, they are considered part of the defense industrial base.
3. House Committee on Armed Services, *Challenges to Doing Business with the Department of Defense: Findings of the Panel on Business Challenges in the Defense Industry,* 48.

CHAPTER 4. A ROMP THROUGH THE EARLY HISTORY OF COMBAT RATIONS

1. R. W. Davies, "The Roman Military Diet," *Britannia* 2 (1971): 135.

CHAPTER 5. DISRUPTIVE INNOVATION: THE TIN CAN

1. Harper Leech and John Charles Carroll, *Armour and His Times* (New York: D. Appleton-Century, 1938), 52.
2. *Report of the Commission Appointed by the President to Investigate the Conduct of the War Department in the War with Spain*, 56th Cong., 1st sess., Sen. Doc. No. 221 (Washington, DC: Government Printing Office, 1899).
3. Ibid., 417.
4. "Eagan Denounces Miles as a Liar: Sensational Attack upon the Army's Commander," *New York Times*, January 13, 1899, 1.
5. *Report of the Commission Appointed by the President to Investigate the Conduct of the War Department in the War with Spain*, 52.
6. Ibid., 156.
7. Ibid., 50.
8. Ibid., 62.

CHAPTER 6. WORLD WAR II, THE SUBSISTENCE LAB, AND ITS MERRY BAND OF INSIDERS

1. George Baker, Frederick A. Brooks, Harold Goss, et al., "Emil Mrak: Faculty Research Lecturer at Davis," *University Bulletin*, vol. 6, no. 15, November 11, 1957.
2. Barbara Moran, "Dinner Goes to War: The Long Battle for Edible Combat Rations Is Finally Being Won," *American Heritage's Invention & Technology* 14, no. 1 (Summer 1998): 10–19.
3. George Bartlett, "Army's Famous 'C' Ration Developer Now Permanent Resident of Snell Isle," *St. Petersburg Times*, December 17, 1951, 17.
4. Backer says, "The National Archives has somewhere between three hundred and six hundred standard archival boxes of specifications, each of which probably had one thousand to five thousand documents. These are the specifications for all Quartermaster projects, so I don't know what percentage [was] food, but it's totally overwhelming." (Interview by the author, October 14, 2014.)
5. Emil M. Mrak, *Emil M. Mrak—A Journey through Three Epochs: Food Prophet, Creative Chancellor, Senior Statesman of Science*, interviewed by A. I. Dickman (Davis: Oral History Program, University Library, University of California, 1974), 108.
6. W. Franklin Dove, "Developing Food Acceptance Research," *Science* 103, no. 2668 (1946): 187–90.
7. Spencer Ante, *Creative Capital: Georges Doriot and the Birth of Venture Capital* (Boston: Harvard Business Press, 2008), 93–94.
8. Ibid., 94.
9. Erna Rich, "The Development of Subsistence," *The Quartermaster Corps: Organization, Supply, and Services*, vol I. United States Army, Washington, DC: 1995. The quotation appears in a footnote citing an April 14, 1944, letter from B. E.

Proctor, chief of the Subsistence Section, Office of the Quartermaster General, to Dr. J. H. White, acting director of the Subsistence Research Laboratory.

10. John Burchard, *Q.E.D: M.I.T. in World War II.* (New York: John Wiley & Sons, 1948), 75.

11. Kellen Backer, "World War II and the Triumph of Industrialized Food" (Ph.D. diss., University of Wisconsin–Madison, 2012), 60.

12. Mrak, *Emil M. Mrak*, 119.

13. Ibid., 110.

14. Ibid., 111–12.

15. Dwight D. Eisenhower, "Memorandum for Directors and Chiefs of War Department General and Special Staff Divisions and Bureaus and the Commanding Generals of the Major Commands: Subject, Scientific and Technological Resources as Military Assets," April 30, 1946, Division of Engineering and Industrial Research (EIR) Records Group and Division of Engineering (ENG) Records Group (in microfiche collection), National Academy of Sciences Archives, Washington, DC.

16. "Army Now Acting on GI 'Grub Gripes,'" *New York Times,* October 13, 1946, 48.

17. Samuel A. Goldblith, "50 Years of Progress in Food Science and Technology: From Art Based on Experience to Technology Based on Science," *Food Technology* 43, no. 9 (1989): 90.

18. "New Unit Formed for Food Studies," *New York Times,* June 4, 1948, 34.

19. Ibid.

20. Ante, *Creative Capital,* 80.

21. Mrak, *Emil M. Mrak,* 120.

CHAPTER 7. WHAT AMERICA RUNS ON

1. "Army Emergency Rations; Official Report of Tests Made with Soldiers in the Field," *New York Times,* November 2, 1902, 8.

2. Franz A. Koehler, *Special Rations for the Armed Forces, 1946–53,* QMC Historical Studies, series 2, no. 6 (Washington, DC: Historical Branch, Office of the Quartermaster General, 1958).

3. Tim Haslam, *Stars and Stripes and Shadows: How I Remember Vietnam* (Google eBook, 2007), 196.

4. Hershey press releases as cited by Joël Glenn Brenner in *The Emperors of Chocolate: Inside the Secret World of Hershey and Mars* (New York: Random House, 1999), 13.

5. "World Population Data Sheet 2013," Population Reference Bureau, accessed August 4, 2014. http://www.prb.org/Publications/Datasheets/2013/2013-world -population-data-sheet/world-map.aspx#map/world/population/2013.

6. Stephen M. Moody, "Chow Time: Military Feeding from Bunker Hill to Bosnia: The History of the Development and Utilization of Military Rations in the United States Armed Forces" (master's thesis, Kansas State University, 2000), 46–47.

7. Ibid.

8. At the time, Natick had no funds for basic research, so it had enlisted the help of the National Institutes of Health, to which sponsorship of Karel's study is attributed in the 1963 MIT report *Exploration in Future Food-Processing Techniques.*

9. T. P. Labuza, S. R. Tannenbaum, and M. Karel, "Water Content and Stability of Low-Moisture and Intermediate Moisture Foods," *Food Technology* 24 (1970): 543.

10. "Astronauts, Homemakers to Benefit from UM Food Research," press release, University of Minnesota, July 23, 1971.

11. Eric M. Jones, "Drilling Troubles," Corrected Transcript and Commentary, Apollo 15 Lunar Surface Journal, 1996.

CHAPTER 8. HOW DO YOU WANT THAT CHUNKED AND FORMED RESTRUCTURED STEAK?

1. American Cancer Society, *Cancer Facts & Figures 2013*. http://www.cancer.org/research/cancerfactsfigures/cancerfactsfigures/cancer-facts-figures-2013, accessed August 14, 2014.

2. James Plumptre, *The experienced butcher: shewing the respectability and usefulness of his calling, the religious considerations arising from it, the laws relating to it, and various profitable suggestions for the rightly carrying it on: designed not only for the use of butchers, but also for families and readers in general* (London: Printed for Darton, Harvey, and Darton, 1816), 163.

3. Andrew McNamara, "Beef—without Bones," *Army Information Digest* 1-2 (1946): 38.

CHAPTER 9. A LOAF OF EXTENDED-LIFE BREAD, A HUNK OF PROCESSED CHEESE, AND THOU

1. John Croese, Soraya T. Gaze, and Alex Loukas, "Changed Gluten Immunity in Celiac Disease by *Necator americanus* Provides New Insights into Autoimmunity," *International Journal for Parasitology* 43, no. 3–4 (2013): 275–82.

2. William F. Ross and Charles F. Romanus, *The Quartermaster Corps: Operations in the War against Germany*, U.S. Army in World War II (1965; repr., Washington, DC: United States Army, 1991), 145.

3. Advisory Board on Quartermaster Research and Development, Committee on Foods, Quartermaster Food and Container Institute for the Armed Forces, *Yeast: Its Characteristics, Growth, and Function in Baked Products: A Symposium* (Chicago: Department of the Army, 1957), 22.

4. Jack H. Mitchell Jr. and Norbert J. Leinen, eds. *Chemistry of Natural Food Flavors: A Symposium Sponsored by the National Academy of Sciences, National Research Council for the Quartermaster Food and Container Institute for the Armed Forces and Pioneering Research Division*. Natick, MA: Quartermaster Research & Engineering Center, 1957.

5. Irwin Stone, Retarding the staling of bakery products, U.S. Patent 2,615,810A, filed March 4, 1948, and issued October 28, 1952.

6. "Major Research Contributions from the Department of Grain Science and Industry to the Field of Grain Science and Grain Processing," Final Report, Kansas State University, June 30, 2010. www.grains.k-state.edu/doc/centennial -documents/major-research-contributions.pdf, accessed April 17, 2014.

7. J. Y. Kang, A. H. Y. Kang, A. Green, K. A. Gwee, and K. Y. Ho, "Systematic Review: Worldwide Variation in the Frequency of Coeliac Disease and Changes over Time," *Alimentary Pharmacology & Therapeutics* 38, no. 3 (2013): 226–45.

8. As quoted in John H. Perkins, "Reshaping Technology in Wartime: The Effect of Military Goals on Entomological Research and Insect-Control Practices," *Technology and Culture* 19, no. 2 (1978): 169–86.

9. George P. Sanders, "Method of treating cheese," U.S. Patent 2,401,320A, issued June 4, 1946. Cheese dehydration had been performed successfully on skim-milk cheese, such as Parmesan, or by first blending the cheese with water and emulsifiers.

10. "Surplus Sale Rise Put at $23,831,000," *New York Times,* November 19, 1945, 27.

11. Kaleta Doolin, *Fritos® Pie: Stories, Recipes, and More* (College Station: Texas A&M University Press, 2011), 52.

CHAPTER 10. PLASTIC PACKAGING REMODELS THE PLANET

1. U.S. Energy Information Administration, *Annual Energy Review,* 2009. eia.gov/ totalenergy/data/annual/, accessed June 2, 2014.

2. As cited by Graeme K. Hunter in *Vital Forces: The Discovery of the Molecular Basis of Life,* vol. 945 (San Diego: Academic Press, 2000), 180.

3. Hugh W. Field, "New Products of the Petroleum Industry," *Journal of the Franklin Institute* 243, no. 2 (1947): 95–116.

4. Herman Mark, interview by James J. Bohning and Jeffrey L. Sturchio at Polytechnic University, Brooklyn, New York, February 3, March 17, and June 20, 1986, oral history transcript #0030, Chemical Heritage Foundation, Philadelphia, 54–55.

5. Ibid., 58.

6. "Status of Subcontracts under Prime Contract OEMsr-1055," U.S. Army Quartermaster Corps, April 12, 1944.

7. Bruno H. Zimm, interview by James J. Bohning at Anaheim, California, September 9, 1986, oral history transcript #0055, Chemical Heritage Foundation, Philadelphia, 24.

8. "Saran Wrap, Marking 40 Years in Use, Began as Lab Byproduct," *Toledo Blade,* January 25, 1994, 19.

9. Louis C. Rubens, interview by James J. Bohning at Midland, Michigan, August 19, 1986, oral history transcript #0048, Chemical Heritage Foundation, Philadelphia, 8.

10. Raymond F. Boyer, "Herman Mark and the Plastics Industry," *Journal of Polymer Science Part C: Polymer Symposia* 12, no. 1 (1966): 111–18.

11. National Research Council, Advisory Board on Quartermaster Research and Development, minutes of meeting no. 3, June 3, 1949, Division of Engineering (ENG) Records Group, National Academy of Sciences Archives, Washington, DC.

12. E. F. Izard, "Introduction to Symposium on Plasticizers," *Journal of Polymer Science* 2, no. 2 (1947): 11314.

13. Advisory Board on Quartermaster Research and Development, minutes of meeting no. 3.

14. Raymond F. Boyer, Vinylidene chloride compositions stable to light, U.S. Patent 2,429,155A, filed May 4, 1945, and issued October 14, 1947.

15. Saran-Wrap print ad, Dow Chemical Company, 1953.

16. Raymond F. Boyer, interview by James J. Bohning at Michigan Molecular Institute, Midland, Michigan, January 14 and August 19, 1986, oral history transcript #0015, Chemical Heritage Foundation, Philadelphia, 24.

17. Zimm, interview by Bohning, oral history transcript #0055, 24.

18. Advisory Board on Quartermaster Research and Development, minutes of meeting no. 3.

19. Marcus Karel and Gerald Wogan, "Migration of Substances from Flexible Containers for Heat-Processed Foods." Cambridge, MA: Division of Sponsored Research, Massachusetts Institute of Technology, 1962, 16.

20. Rebecca Osvath, "Package Adhesives Must Be Sufficient Barrier, FDA Says," *Food Chemical News* 44, no. 12 (2002): 28.

21. Code of Federal Regulations, Title 21, Food and Drugs, Part 170, Food Additives, as revised April 1, 2013.

22. R. Hauser, J. D. Meeker, N. P. Singh, M. J. Silva, L. Ryan, S. Duty, and A. M. Calafat, "DNA Damage in Human Sperm Is Related to Urinary Levels of Phthalate Monoester and Oxidative Metabolites," *Human Reproduction* 22, no. 3 (2006): 688–95.

23. P. Factor-Litvak, B. Insel, A. M. Calafat, X. Liu, F. Perera, V. A. Rauh, and R. M. Whyatt, "Persistent Associations between Maternal Prenatal Exposure to Phthalates on Child IQ at Age 7 Years," *PLoS One*, December 10, 2014.

24. M. Aznar, M. Canellas, and E. Gaspar, "Migration from Food Packaging Laminates Based on Polyurethane," *Italian Journal of Food Science* 23, SI (2011): 95–98.

25. Du Yeon Bang, Hyung Sik Kim, Bu Young Jung, Min Ji Kim, Minji Kyung, Byung Mu Lee, Youngkwan Lee, et al. "Human Risk Assessment of Endocrine-Disrupting Chemicals Derived from Plastic Food Containers." *Comprehensive Reviews in Food Science and Food Safety* 11, no. 5 (2012): 453–70.

26. Timothy V. Duncan, "Applications of Nanotechnology in Food Packaging and Food Safety: Barrier Materials, Antimicrobials and Sensors," *Journal of Colloid and Interface Science* 363, no. 1 (2011): 1–24.

27. U.S. Food and Drug Administration, "Considering Whether an FDA-Regulated Product Involves the Application of Nanotechnology: Guidance for Industry," June 2014.

CHAPTER 11. LATE-NIGHT MUNCHIES? BREAK OUT THE THREE-YEAR-OLD PIZZA AND MONTHS-OLD GUACAMOLE

1. Marcus Cato, *De agricultura*, Loeb Classical Library. Translated by W. D. Hooper and H. B. Ash. (Cambridge, MA: Harvard University Press, 1934), 162.
2. Lothar Leistner and Grahame W. Gould, *Hurdle Technologies: Combination Treatments for Food Stability, Safety and Quality* (Medford, MA: Springer Science & Business Media, 2002), 44.
3. H. Roger, "Action des hautes pressions sur quelques bacteries," *Comptes rendus hebdomadaires des séances de l'Académie des Sciences*, 1895, 963–65.
4. http://www.marlerblog.com/files/2013/01/Odwalla2.png, accessed October 1, 2014.
5. Science Board to the U.S. Food and Drug Administration, Advisory Committee meeting transcript, October 21, 1998, 41–42.

CHAPTER 12. SUPERMARKET TOUR

1. "Fliers May Prepare Meal in One Minute," *Washington Post*, June 23, 1947, 2.
2. *Radiation Sterilization of Food: Hearing Before the Subcommittee on Research and Development of the Joint Committee on Atomic Energy*, 84th Cong. 37 (May 9, 1955).
3. Nicholas Buchanan, "The Atomic Meal: The Cold War and Irradiated Foods, 1945–1963," *History and Technology: An International Journal* 21, no. 2 (2005): 221–49.
4. "The Road to Irradiation Breakthroughs," *Executive Intelligence Review* 12, no. 48 (1985): 22–27.
5. Advisory Board on Military Personnel Supplies, Division of Engineering— National Research Council, minutes of meeting, July 28–29, 1968, Division of Engineering (ENG) Records Group, National Academy of Sciences Archives, Washington, DC.
6. National Academy of Sciences–National Research Council, Advisory Board on Quartermaster Research and Development, Committee on Foods, Subcommittee on Fruits and Vegetables, minutes of meeting, June 21, 1951, Division of Engineering (ENG) Records Group, National Academy of Sciences Archives, Washington, DC.
7. George Kent, "Two Practical Men Revolutionize the Processing of Rice," *Washington Post*, January 16, 1944, B6.
8. Aaron Karp, "FAA: US Commercial Aircraft Fleet Shrank in 2011," *Air Transport World*, March 12, 2012, accessed October 26, 2014. http://atwonline.com/aircraft-amp-engines/faa-us-commercial-aircraft-fleet-shrank-2011.
9. Paul A. Lachance, interview by Jennifer Ross-Nazzal, Houston, Texas, and New Brunswick, New Jersey, May 4, 2006, NASA Johnson Space Center Oral History Project, accessed October 25, 2014. http://www.jsc.nasa.gov/history/oral_histories/LachancePA/LachancePA_5-4-06.htm.
10. Margaret Mead, "The Factor of Food Habits," in "Nutrition and Food Supply: The War and After," *Annals of the American Academy of Political and Social Science* 225 (1943): 136–41.

CHAPTER 13. COMING UP NEXT FROM THE HOUSE OF GI JOE

1. Spencer Ante, *Creative Capital: Georges Doriot and the Birth of Venture Capital* (Boston: Harvard Business Press, 2008), 80.
2. David H. Hsa and Martin Kenney, "Organizing Venture Capital: The Rise and Demise of American Research & Development Corporation, 1946–1973," working paper of the Wharton School, University of Pennsylvania, and the University of California at Davis, 2004, 37.
3. Massachusetts Institute of Technology, Proctor Papers, MC 0268, Institute Archives and Special Collections, MIT Libraries, Cambridge, MA.
4. Emil M. Mrak, *Emil M. Mrak—A Journey through Three Epochs: Food Prophet, Creative Chancellor, Senior Statesman of Science*, interviewed by A. I. Dickman (Davis: Oral History Program, University Library, University of California, 1974), 115–16.
5. Dietary Supplement Health and Education Act of 1994, 108 Stat. 4325-4335, 103rd Cong. (Oct. 25, 1994).
6. Ann H. Barrett and Armand Vincent Cardello, *Military Food Engineering and Ration Technology* (Lancaster, PA: DEStech Publications, 2012), 278.
7. Ibid., 276.
8. "Development of a Phage-Based Technology for Eliminating or Significantly Reducing Contamination of Fruits and Vegetables with *E. coli* O157:H7," Intralytix, press release, November 26, 2008.
9. "Intralytix Receives FDA Regulatory Clearance for Phage-Based *E. coli* Technology," Intralytix, press release, February 8, 2011.
10. Army Environmental Policy Institute, *Use of Renewable Energy in Contingency Operations* (Arlington, VA: Army Environmental Policy Institute, March 2007), 8–9.

CHAPTER 14. DO WE REALLY WANT OUR CHILDREN EATING LIKE SPECIAL OPS?

1. "Housewife of Future May Cook Only as Hobby," *Palm Beach Daily News*, January 13, 1956, 6.
2. Ann H. Barrett and Armand Vincent Cardello, *Military Food Engineering and Ration Technology* (Lancaster, PA: DEStech Publications, 2012), xiii.
3. Tom Neltner and Maricel Maffini, "Generally Recognized as Secret: Chemicals Added to Food in the United States," report by the Natural Resources Defense Council, April 2014. www.nrdc.org/food/files/safety-loophole-for-chemicals-in-food-report.pdf, accessed December 31, 2014.

Selected Sources

Below is a partial list of the sources used in writing this book. A complete list may be found at www.anastaciamarxdesalcedo.com.

USED THROUGHOUT THE BOOK

Advisory Board on Military Personnel Supplies. Meeting notes and reports, 1966–1982. Division of Engineering (ENG) Records Group. National Academy of Sciences Archives, Washington, DC.

Advisory Board on Quartermaster Research and Development, National Research Council. Meeting notes and reports, 1949–1965. Division of Engineering (ENG) Records Group. National Academy of Sciences Archives, Washington, DC.

Barrett, Ann H., and Armand Vincent Cardello. *Military Food Engineering and Ration Technology.* Lancaster, PA: DEStech Publications, 2012.

Committee on Quartermaster Problems. Meeting notes and reports, 1942–1948. Division of Engineering and Industrial Research (EIR) Records Group. National Academy of Sciences Archives, Washington, DC.

Darsch, Gerard. Multiple interviews by the author, March and April 2014.

Division of Engineering and Industrial Research (EIR) Records Group and Division of Engineering (ENG) Records Group (in microfiche collection). National Academy of Sciences Archives, Washington, DC.

Lund, Daryl. Interview by the author, July 8, 2014.

McGee, Harold. *On Food and Cooking: The Science and Lore of the Kitchen.* Completely rev. and updated ed. New York: Scribner, 2004.

Shephard, Sue. *Pickled, Potted, and Canned: The Story of Food Preserving.* London: Headline, 2000.

U.S. Army Quartermaster Corps. Meeting notes and reports, various committees, 1950s. Division of Engineering and Industrial Research (EIR) Records Group and Division of Engineering (ENG) Records Group. National Academy of Sciences Archives, Washington, DC.

CHAPTER 2. AMERICAN FOOD SYSTEM, CENTRAL COMMAND, PART ONE

U.S. Army Natick Soldier Research, Development and Engineering Center, site visits by the author in February and March 2011.

CHAPTER 3. AMERICAN FOOD SYSTEM, CENTRAL COMMAND, PART TWO

Allen, Joe. "A Long, Hard Journey: From Bayh-Dole to the Federal Technology Transfer Act." *Journal of the Association of University Technology Managers* 1, no. 1 (2009): 21–32.

American Association for the Advancement of Science. *AAAS Report XXXIII: Research and Development FY 2009.* Washington, DC: American Association for the Advancement of Science, 2008.

Berteau, David, Guy Ben-Ari, Jesse Ellman, Reed Livergood, David Morrow, and Gregory Sanders. *Defense Contract Trends. U.S. Department of Defense Contract Spending and the Supporting Industrial Base: An Annotated Brief.* Washington, DC: Center for Strategic and International Studies, 2011.

Boroush, Mark. E-mail correspondence with the author, November and December, 2012.

Chang, Ike Yi, Steven Galing, Carolyn Wong, Howell Yee, Elliot I. Axelband, Mark Onesi, and Kenneth P. Horn. *Use of Public-Private Partnerships to Meet Future Army Needs.* Santa Monica, CA: Rand, 1999.

Cohen, Wesley M., and Stephen A. Merrill, eds. *Patents in the Knowledge-Based Economy.* Washington, DC: National Academies Press, 2003.

Division of Science Resources Statistics, National Science Foundation. *Federal Funds for Research and Development: Fiscal Years 2007–09.* Arlington, VA: Division of Science Resources Statistics, National Science Foundation, 2010.

Division of Science Resources Statistics, National Science Foundation. *Federal R&D Funding by Budget Function: Fiscal Years 2007–09.* Arlington, VA: Division of Science Resources Statistics, National Science Foundation, 2008.

Fountain, Augustus Way, III. "Transforming Defense Basic Research Strategy." The U.S. Army Professional Writing Collection. Accessed November 12, 2013. http://strategicstudiesinstitute.army.mil/pubs/parameters/Articles/04winter/fountain.pdf.

Gonsalves, Cynthia. Interview by the author, September 27, 2012.

Halchin, L. Elaine. *Other Transaction (OT) Authority.* CRS Report No. RL34760. Washington, DC: Congressional Research Service, Library of Congress, 2008.

House Committee on Armed Services. *Challenges to Doing Business with the Department of Defense: Findings of the Panel on Business Challenges in the Defense Industry.* Washington, DC, March 19, 2012.

Hughes, Mary Elizabeth, Susannah Vale Howieson, Gina Walejko, Nayanee Gupta, Seth Jonas, Ashley T. Brenner, Dawn Holmes, Edward Shyu, and Stephanie Shipp. *Technology Transfer and Commercialization Landscape of the Federal Laboratories.* Washington, DC: Institute for Defense Analyses, Science and Technology Policy Institute, 2011.

Kennedy, Donald. "Industry and Academia in Transition." *Science* 302, no. 5649 (2003): 1293.

Moteff, John D. *Defense Research: A Primer on the Department of Defense's Research, Development, Test and Evaluation (RDT&E) Program.* Fort Belvoir, VA: Defense Technical Information Center, 1999.

National Center for Science and Engineering Statistics, National Science Foundation. *National Patterns of R&D Resources: 2009 Data Update.* Washington, DC: National Center for Science and Engineering Statistics, National Science Foundation, 2012.

Schacht, Wendy H. *Industrial Competitiveness and Technological Advancement Debate Over Government Policy.* CRS Report No. RL33528. Washington, DC: Congressional Research Service, Library of Congress, 2012.

Schaffner, Donald. Interview by the author, September 4, 2014.

"Solicitation No: SP0300-02-R-4030, Spokane, Washington and Idaho Regions." https://www.troopsupport.dla.mil/subs/pv/regions/west/4030.pdf.

U.S. Army Natick Soldier Research, Development and Engineering Center. *How to Do Business with the NSRDEC Guidebook.* Natick, MA: U.S. Army Natick Soldier Research, Development and Engineering Center, 2011.

Watts, Barry, and Todd Harrison. *Sustaining Critical Sectors of the U.S. Defense Industrial Base.* Washington, DC: Center for Strategic and Budgetary Assessments, 2011.

Wells, Linton, II, and Samuel Bendett. "Public-Private Cooperation in the Department of Defense: A Framework for Analysis and Recommendations for Action." *Defense Horizons* 74 (2012): 1–12.

Wong, Carolyn. *An Analysis of Collaborative Research Opportunities for the Army.* Santa Monica, CA: Rand, 1998.

Yamaner, Michael. E-mail correspondence with the author, November 2012.

CHAPTER 4. A ROMP THROUGH THE EARLY HISTORY OF COMBAT RATIONS

Bezeczky, Támas. "Amphora Inscriptions—Legionary Supply." *Britannia* 27 (1996): 329–36.

Carrasco, Davíd. "Give Me Some Skin: The Charisma of the Aztec Warrior." In "Meso-american Religions. A Special Issue on the Occasion of the Seventeenth International Congress of the History of Religions, Mexico City, August 5–12, 1995." *History of Religions* 35, no. 1 (1995): 1–26.

Dalby, Andrew. "Greeks Abroad: Social Organisation and Food among the Ten Thousand." *Journal of Hellenic Studies* 112 (1992): 16–30.

Davies, R. W. "The Roman Military Diet." *Britannia* 2 (1971): 122–42.

The Electronic Text Corpus of Sumerian Literature. "Dumuzid and Enkimdu: translation." Accessed June 14, 2012. http://etcsl.orinst.ox.ac.uk/section4/tr40833.htm.

Fernández-Jalvo, Yolanda, J. Carlos Diez, Isabel Cáceres, and Jordi Rosell. "Human Cannibalism in the Early Pleistocene of Europe." *Journal of Human Evolution* 37, no. 3–4 (1999): 591–622.

Figueira, Thomas J. "Mess Contributions and Subsistence at Sparta." *Transactions of the American Philological Association* 114 (1984): 87–109.

Flacelière, Robert. *Daily Life in Greece at the Time of Pericles.* Translated by Peter Green. New York: Macmillan, 1965.

France, John. "Close Order and Close Quarter: The Culture of Combat in the West." *International History Review* 27, no. 3 (2005): 498–517.

Frost, Frank. "Sausage and Meat Preservation in Antiquity." *Greek, Roman, and Byzantine Studies* 40 (1999): 241–52.

Gabriel, Richard A. *The Great Armies of Antiquity.* Westport, CT: Praeger, 2002.

Harner, Michael. "The Ecological Basis for Aztec Sacrifice." American *Ethnologist* 4, no. 1 (1977): 117–35.

Holmes, Bob. "Manna or Millstone: Why Would Anyone Swap a Life of Hunting and Gathering to Start Farming? There Was More to It Than Filling Bellies." *New Scientist* 183, no. 2465 (2004): 29–31.

Ortiz de Montellano, Bernard R. "Aztec Cannibalism: An Ecological Necessity?" *Science* 200, no. 4342 (1978): 611–17.

Pickstone, Joan E. "Roman Cookery." *Greece & Rome* 4, no. 12 (1935): 168–74.

Pinker, Steven. *The Blank Slate: The Modern Denial of Human Nature.* New York: Viking, 2003.

Standage, Tom. *An Edible History of Humanity.* New York: Walker & Company, 2009.

Stoneking, Mark. "Widespread Prehistoric Human Cannibalism: Easier to Swallow?" *Trends in Ecology & Evolution* 18, no. 10 (2003): 489–90.

Swatland, H. J. *Meat Cuts and Muscle Foods.* Nottingham, UK: Nottingham University Press, 2004.

Tannahill, Reay. *Food in History.* New York: Three Rivers Press, 1988.

Thadeusz, Frank. "Alcohol's Neolithic Origins: Brewing Up a Civilization." *Spiegel Online*, December 24, 2009.

Walker, Phillip L. "A Bioarchaeological Perspective on the History of Violence." *Annual Review of Anthropology* 30 (2001): 573–96.

Wilson, Edward O. *The Social Conquest of Earth.* New York: Liveright, 2012.

Wrangham, Richard. *Catching Fire: How Cooking Made Us Human.* New York: Basic Books, 2009.

CHAPTER 5. DISRUPTIVE INNOVATION: THE TIN CAN

Adiba, Sandrine, Clément Nizak, Minus van Baalen, Erick Denamur, and Frantz Depaulis. "From Grazing Resistance to Pathogenesis: The Coincidental Evolution of Virulence Factors." *PLoS One*, August 11, 2010.

Anderson, W. A., P. J. McClure, A. C. Baird-Parker, and M. B. Cole. "The Application of a Log-Logistic Model to Describe the Thermal Inactivation of *Clostridium botulinum* 213B at Temperatures Below 121.1°C." *Journal of Applied Bacteriology* 80, no. 3 (1996): 283–90.

Appert, Nicolas. *The Book for All Households; or, The Art of Preserving Animal and Vegetable Substances for Many Years.* Translated by K. G. Bitting. Chicago: Glass Container Association of America, 1920.

Aziz, Ramy. "The Case for Biocentric Microbiology." *Gut Pathogens* 1, no. 1 (2009): 16.

Beede, Benjamin R. *The War of 1898 and U.S. Interventions, 1898–1934: An Encyclopedia.* New York: Routledge, 1994.

Bengmark, S. "Advanced Glycation and Lipoxidation End Products—Amplifiers of Inflammation: The Role of Food." *Journal of Parenteral and Enteral Nutrition* 31, no. 5 (2007): 430–40.

Bennett, J. W., and M. Klich. "Mycotoxins." *Clinical Microbiology Reviews* 16, no. 3 (2003): 497–516.

Boeger, Palmer Henry. "Hardtack and Coffee: The Commissary Department, 1861–1865." Ph.D. diss., University of Wisconsin, 1953.

Brown, Sam P., Daniel M. Cornforth, and Nicole Mideo. "Evolution of Virulence in Opportunistic Pathogens: Generalism, Plasticity, and Control." *Trends in Microbiology* 20, no. 7 (2012): 336–42.

Cano, R., and M. Borucki. "Revival and Identification of Bacterial Spores in 25- to 40-Million-Year-Old Dominican Amber." *Science* 268, no. 5213 (1995): 1060–64.

Cénat, Jean-Philippe. "De la guerre de siège à la guerre de mouvement: Une révolution logistique à l'époque de la Révolution et de l'Empire?" *Annales historiques de la Révolution Française* 348 (2007): 101–15.

Center for Food Safety and Applied Nutrition, U.S. Food and Drug Administration. *Bad Bug Book: Foodborne Pathogenic Microorganisms and Natural Toxins Handbook.* 2nd ed. McLean, VA: Center for Food Safety and Applied Nutrition, U.S. Food and Drug Administration, 2012.

Ceuppens, Siele, Mieke Uyttendaele, Katrien Drieskens, Andreja Rajkovic, Nico Boon, and Tom Van de Wiele. "Survival of *Bacillus cereus* Vegetative Cells and Spores during In Vitro Simulation of Gastric Passage." *Journal of Food Protection* 75, no. 4 (2012): 690–94.

Cook, Charles K. "The Glass Beverage Bottles of the HMS St. George: 1785-1811." Master's thesis. University of Southern Denmark, September 2012.

Croddy, Eric A., James J. Wirtz, and Jeffrey A. Larsen, eds. *Weapons of Mass Destruction: An Encyclopedia of Worldwide Policy, Technology, and History.* Santa Barbara, CA: ABC-CLIO, 2005.

Davis, Eugenia A. "Functionality of Sugars: Physicochemical Interactions in Foods." *American Journal of Clinical Nutrition* 62, no. 1 (1995): 170–77S.

Day, Ivan. "The Art of Confectionery." http://www.historicfood.com/The%20Art%20of%20confectionery.pdf.

Deák, Tibor. *Handbook of Food Spoilage Yeasts.* 2nd ed. Boca Raton, FL: CRC Press, 2007.

Donnenberg, Michael S., and Thomas S. Whittam. "Pathogenesis and Evolution of Virulence in Enteropathogenic and Enterohemorrhagic *Escherichia coli.*" *Journal of Clinical Investigation* 107, no. 5 (2001): 539–48.

Ercolini, D., F. Russo, A. Nasi, P. Ferranti, and F. Villani. "Mesophilic and Psychrotrophic Bacteria from Meat and Their Spoilage Potential In Vitro and in Beef." *Applied and Environmental Microbiology* 75, no. 7 (2009): 1990–2001.

Franzetti, Laura, and Mauro Scarpellini. "Characterisation of *Pseudomonas spp.* Isolated from Foods." *Annals of Microbiology* 57, no. 1 (2007): 39–47.

Fuchs, Thilo M., Wolfgang Eisenreich, Jürgen Heesemann, and Werner Goebel. "Metabolic Adaptation of Human Pathogenic and Related Nonpathogenic Bacteria to Extra- and Intracellular Habitats." *FEMS Microbiology Reviews* 36, no. 2 (2012): 43562.

Garzón, León. "Microbial Life and Temperature: A Semi Empirical Approach." *Origins of Life and Evolution of the Biosphere* 34, no. 4 (2004): 421–38.

German, J. Bruce. "Food Processing and Lipid Oxidation." *Advances in Experimental Medicine and Biology* 459 (1999): 23–50.

Hedayati, M. T., A. C. Pasqualotto, P. A. Warn, P. Bowyer, and D. W. Denning. "*Aspergillus flavus:* Human Pathogen, Allergen and Mycotoxin Producer." *Microbiology* 153, no. 6 (2007): 1677–92.

Kanner, Joseph. "Dietary Advanced Lipid Oxidation Endproducts Are Risk Factors to Human Health." *Molecular Nutrition & Food Research* 51, no. 9 (2007): 1094–101.

Levin, Bruce. "The Evolution and Maintenance of Virulence in Microparasites." *Emerging Infectious Diseases* 2, no. 2 (1996): 93–102.

Martins, Sara, Wim Jongen, and Martinus van Boekel. "A Review of Maillard Reaction in Food and Implications to Kinetic Modelling." *Trends in Food Science & Technology* 11, no. 9–10 (2000): 364–73.

Massiallot, François. *Nouvelle instruction pour les confitures, les liqueurs, et les fruits.* Paris, 1692.

Naila, Aishath, Steve Flint, Graham Fletcher, Phil Bremer, and Gerrit Meerdink. "Control of Biogenic Amines in Food—Existing and Emerging Approaches." *Journal of Food Science* 75, no. 7 (2010): R139–50.

Nataro, James P., and James B. Kaper. "Diarrheagenic *Escherichia coli.*" *Clinical Microbiology Reviews* 11, no. 1 (1998): 142–201.

Pitt, John I., and Ailsa D. Hocking. *Fungi and Food Spoilage.* 3rd ed. New York: Springer, 2009.

Popoff, M. R. "Multifaceted Interactions of Bacterial Toxins with the Gastrointestinal Mucosa." *Future Microbiology* 6, no. 7 (2011): 763–97.

Ranson, Edward. "Nelson A. Miles as Commanding General, 1895–1903." *Military Affairs* 39 (1966): 179–200.

Ray, Bibek, and Arun K. Bhunia. *Fundamental Food Microbiology.* 3rd ed. Boca Raton, FL: CRC Press, 2004.

Report of the Commission Appointed by the President to Investigate the Conduct of the War Department in the War with Spain. 56th Cong., 1st sess., Sen. Doc. No. 221. Washington, DC: Government Printing Office, 1899.

Rizzi, George P. "Free Radicals in the Maillard Reaction." *Food Reviews International* 19, no. 4 (2003): 375–95.

Ruiz-Capillas, Claudia, and Francisco Jiménez-Colmenero. "Biogenic Amines in Meat and Meat Products." *Critical Reviews in Food Science and Nutrition* 44 (2004): 489–99.

Sawires, Y. S., and J. G. Songer. "*Clostridium perfringens:* Insight into Virulence Evolution and Population Structure." *Anaerobe* 12, no. 1 (2006): 23–43.

Silva, Manuel T. "Classical Labeling of Bacterial Pathogens According to Their Lifestyle in the Host: Inconsistencies and Alternatives." *Frontiers in Microbiology* 3, no. 71 (2012).

Skirbunt, Peter D. *The Illustrated History of American Military Commissaries.* Vol. 1, *The Defense Commissary Agency and Its Predecessors, 1775–1988.* Fort Lee, VA: Office of Corporate Communications, Defense Commissary Agency, 2008.

Souza dos Reis, Roberta, and Fabiana Horn. "Enteropathogenic *Escherichia coli, Samonella, Shigella* and *Yersinia:* Cellular Aspects of Host-Bacteria Interactions in Enteric Diseases." *Gut Pathogens* 2, no. 1 (2010): 8.

Sperber, William H., and Michael P. Doyle, eds. *Compendium of the Microbiological Spoilage of Food and Beverages.* New York: Springer, 2009.

Staum, Martin S. "The Enlightenment Transformed: The Institute Prize Contests." *Eighteenth-Century Studies* 19, no. 2 (1985–86): 153–79.

Stenfors Arnesen, Lotte P., Annette Fagerlund, and Per Einar Granum. "From Soil to Gut: *Bacillus cereus* and Its Food Poisoning Toxins." *FEMS Microbiology Reviews* 32, no. 4 (2008): 579–606.

Tielens, A. G. G. M. *The Physics and Chemistry of the Interstellar Medium.* Cambridge: Cambridge University Press, 2005.

Tucker, Spencer, ed. *The Encyclopedia of the Spanish-American and Philippine-American Wars: A Political, Social, and Military History.* Vol. 1: A–L. Santa Barbara, CA: ABC-CLIO, 2009.

Weeks, Benjamin S. *Alcamo's Microbes and Society.* Sudbury, MA: Jones & Bartlett, 2011.

Wilson, Bee. *Swindled: The Dark History of Food Fraud, from Poisoned Candy to Counterfeit Coffee.* Princeton, NJ: Princeton University Press, 2008.

Wilson, Mark. E-mail correspondence with the author, January 2012.

Winfield, M. D., and E. A. Groisman. "Role of Nonhost Environments in the Lifestyles of *Salmonella* and *Escherichia coli.*" *Applied and Environmental Microbiology* 69, no. 7 (2003): 3687–94.

Wright, Brian D. "The Economics of Invention Incentives: Patents, Prizes, and Research Contracts." *American Economic Review* 73, no. 4 (1983): 691–707.

Xayarath, Bobbi, and Nancy E. Freitag. "Optimizing the Balance Between Host and Environmental Survival Skills: Lessons Learned from *Listeria monocytogenes.*" *Future Microbiology* 7, no. 7 (2012): 838–52.

CHAPTER 6. WORLD WAR II, THE SUBSISTENCE LAB, AND ITS MERRY BAND OF INSIDERS

Ante, Spencer. *Creative Capital: Georges Doriot and the Birth of Venture Capital.* Boston: Harvard Business Press, 2008.

Backer, Kellen. Interview by the author, October 14, 2014.

———. "World War II and the Triumph of Industrialized Food." Ph.D. diss., University of Wisconsin–Madison, 2012.

"Biographical Sketch of Col. Rohland A. Isker." Fort Lee, VA: Army Quartermaster Museum, nd.: 22–25.

Buchanan, Nicholas. "The Atomic Meal: The Cold War and Irradiated Foods, 1945–1963." *History and Technology* 21, no. 2 (2005): 221–49.

Burchard, John. *Q.E.D: M.I.T. in World War II.* Cambridge, MA: Technology Press, 1948.

Bureau of the Census. *Personnel and Pay of the Military Branch of the Federal Government: 1934 to 1945.* Washington, DC, 1946.

"Celebrating the 50th Anniversary of the Institute of Food Technologists." *Food Technology* (September 1989): 1–168.

Doriot, Georges. "Research in the Military Planning Division, Quartermaster Corps." *Journal of Applied Physics* 16, no. 4 (1945): 235.

Eisenhower, Dwight. "Memorandum for Directors and Chiefs of War Department, General and Special Staff Divisions and Bureaus and the Commanding General of the Major Commands." April 30, 1946. Division of Engineering and Industrial Research (EIR) Records Group and Division of Engineering (ENG) Records Group (in microfiche collection). National Academy of Sciences Archives, Washington, DC.

Feeney, Robert, Eldon Askew, and Deborah Jezior. "The Development and Evolution of U.S. Army Field Rations." *Nutrition Reviews* 53, no. 8 (1995): 221–25.

"Food Research Unit Is Organized by Army: Board to Develop New Products and Rations." *New York Times,* December 26, 1942, 16.

"The Food Technology Conference at the Massachusetts Institute of Technology." *Science,* June 2, 1939, 2318.

Gelman, George. "Committee on Food Research." *Oil & Soap* 23, no. 12 (1946): 389–91.

Goldblith, Samuel. "50 Years of Progress in Food Science and Technology: From Art Based on Experience to Technology Based on Science." *Food Technology* (September 1989): 9.

———. *Of Microbes and Molecules: Food Technology, Nutrition, and Applied Biology at M.I.T., 1873–1988.* Trumbull, CT: Food and Nutrition Press, 1995.

Gupta, Udayan, ed. *The First Venture Capitalist: Georges Doriot on Leadership, Capital, & Business Organization.* Calgary, Canada: Gondolier, 2004.

Hanson, Luther, Interview by the author, May 23, 2014.

Hewlett, Frank. "Troops on Bataan Routed by Malaria. Poor Diet Also a Factor." *New York Times,* April 18, 1942, 5.

"Larger Capital Fund Has Been Formed to Aid New Enterprises." *Boston Globe*, August 9, 1946, 12.

Lightbody, Marcia. "Building a Future: World War II Quartermaster Corps." *Military Review* (January–February 2001): 1.

Massachusetts Institute of Technology, Office of the President, 1944–51. Department of Food Technology, Food Sterilization Building, Quartermaster's Laboratory and Space: Post–World War II Readjustment of Department of Food Technology. AC 0004, boxes 88, 176, and 205. Institute Archives and Special Collections, MIT Libraries, Cambridge, MA.

Miller, Lillian, Frederick Voss, and Jeannette M. Hussey. *The Lazzaroni: Science and Scientists in Mid-Nineteenth-Century America.* Published for the National Portrait Gallery, Smithsonian Institution. Washington, DC: Smithsonian Institution Press, 1972.

Moody, Stephen. Interview by the author, July 9, 2014.

Moran, Barbara. "Dinner Goes to War: The Long Battle for Edible Combat Rations Is Finally Being Won." *American Heritage's Invention & Technology* 14, no. 1 (1998): 10–19.

Mrak, Emil M. *Emil M. Mrak—A Journey through Three Epochs: Food Prophet, Creative Chancellor, Senior Statesman of Science.* Interviewed by A. I. Dickman. Davis: Oral History Program, University Library, University of California, 1974.

———. "A Microbiologist Turned Administrator—How It Happened." *Annual Review of Microbiology* 28, no. 1 (1974): 1–24.

———. "The Role of Chemistry and Technology in the Development of Modern Food." Dedication at Cornell University, Food Research Building, Ithaca, NY, 1960.

———. "75th Anniversary of Opening of Davis Campus." Speech at the University of California, Davis, CA, 1984.

"New Unit Formed for Food Studies: Wartime Container Problems Will Be Objective of Group." *New York Times*, June 4, 1948.

Ohly, John H. *Industrialists in Olive Drab: The Emergency Operation of Private Industries during World War II.* Edited by Clayton D. Laurie. Washington, DC: U.S. Army Center of Military History, 2000.

Oyos, Matthew M. "Theodore Roosevelt, Congress, and the Military: U.S. Civil-Military Relations in the Early Twentieth Century." *Presidential Studies Quarterly* 30, no. 2 (2000): 312–31.

Paarlberg, Robert L. "Knowledge as Power: Science, Military Dominance, and U.S. Security." *International Security* 29, no. 1 (2004): 122–51.

Proctor, Bernard. *Development of the Department of Food Technology at the Massachusetts Institute of Technology and Proposed Program for Future Activities.* Cambridge, MA: Massachusetts Institute of Technology, 1951.

Risch, Erna, and Chester Kieffer. "The Development of Subsistence." In *The Quartermaster Corps: Organization, Supply, and Services*, 2:174–207. Reprint, Washington, DC: U.S. Army Center of Military History, 1988.

Schubert, Frank N. *Mobilization.* Washington, DC: U.S. Army Center of Military History, 1995.

CHAPTER 7. WHAT AMERICA RUNS ON

Barbosa-Cánovas, Gustavo V., Anthony J. Fontana Jr., Shelly J. Schmidt, and Theodore P. Labuza, eds. *Water Activity in Foods: Fundamentals and Applications.* Ames, IA: IFT Press/Blackwell Publishing, 2007.

Bernhardt, Joshua. "Government Control of Sugar during the War." *Quarterly Journal of Economics* 33, no. 4 (1919): 672–713.

Borg, Axel. Interview by the author, June 3, 2014.

Brenner, Joël Glenn. *The Emperors of Chocolate: Inside the Secret World of Hershey and Mars.* New York: Random House, 1999.

Brockmann, Maxwell C. "Development of Intermediate Moisture Foods for Military Use." *Food Technology* 24, no. 8 (1970): 60–64.

Brown, W. C. "The U.S. Army Emergency Ration." *Infantry Journal* 16, no. 2 (1920): 656–60.

Buchanan, Ben F. "General Foods Product Development as Related to Aerospace Food Problems." Speech given at the Space Food Technology Conference, University of South Florida, Tampa, April 15, 1969.

Burgess, Hovey M. Animal food and method of making same. U.S. Patent 3,202,514, filed July 15, 1963, and issued August 24, 1965.

Bustead, R. L., and J. M. Tuomy. "Food Quality Design for Gemini and Apollo Space Programs: Technical Conference Transactions." Natick, MA: U.S. Army Natick Laboratories, 1966.

"Candy Important Element in Army Diet." *Boston Globe,* May 26, 1941, 10.

Committee on Military Nutrition Research, Food and Nutrition Board, Institute of Medicine. "The New Generation Survival Ration." Washington, DC: Committee on Military Nutrition Research, Food and Nutrition Board, Institute of Medicine, 1991.

Connell, Sanjida. *Sugar: The Grass That Changed the World.* London: Virgin, 2004.

Downey, Morgan, and Christopher Still. "Survey of Anti-Obesity Legislation: Are These Laws Working?" *Current Opinion in Endocrinology, Diabetes and Obesity* 19, no. 5 (2012): 375–80.

Durst, Jack Rowland. *All Purpose Matrices for Compressed Food Bars.* Natick, MA: Food Division, U.S. Army Natick Laboratories, 1966.

Dusselier, Jane. "Bonbons, Lemon Drops, and Oh Henry! Bars: Candy, Consumer Culture, and the Construction of Gender, 1895–1920." In *Kitchen Culture in America: Popular Representations of Food, Gender and Race,* edited by Sherrie A. Inness, 13–49. Philadelphia: University of Pennsylvania Press, 2001.

Frear, William. "The Dairy Industry in Pennsylvania." In *Fourteenth Annual Report of the Pennsylvania Department of Agriculture,* 92–101. Harrisburg: Harrisburg Publishing Company, State Printer, 1908.

Gallant, Nanette. "Subsistence in Space." *Quartermaster Professional Bulletin* (Summer 1992). Accessed July 6, 2013. www.qmfound.com/subsistence_in_space.htm.

Goldblith, Samuel A. *Of Microbes and Molecules: Food Technology, Nutrition, and Applied Biology at M.I.T., 1873–1988.* Trumbull, CT: Food and Nutrition Press, 1995.

Gordon, Robert V. "New Food for Third Skylab Mission." Release No. 73-143. Houston, TX: National Aeronautics and Space Administration, 1973.

Gould, Stephen Jay. "Phyletic Size Decrease in Hershey Bars." In *Hen's Teeth and Horse's Toes: Further Reflections in Natural History*, 313–19. New York: W. W. Norton, 1984.

Hewitt, Eric John. *All-Purpose Matrix for Molded Food Bars.* Natick, MA: U.S. Army Material Command, U.S. Army Natick Laboratories, 1965.

Hostetter, Christina J. "Sugar Allies: How Hershey and Coca-Cola Used Government Contracts and Sugar Exemptions to Elude Sugar Rationing Regulations." College Park: University of Maryland, 2004.

Hui, Y. H. *Handbook of Food Science, Technology, and Engineering.* Boca Raton, FL: Taylor & Francis, 2006.

Hundert, Gershon David. *The Yivo Encyclopedia of Jews in Eastern Europe.* New Haven, CT: Yale University Press, 2008.

Karel, Marcus. "Chemical Effects in Food Stored at Room Temperature." *Journal of Chemical Education* 61, no. 4 (1984): 335.

———. E-mail correspondence with the author, 2012–14.

———. "Physical and Chemical Considerations in Freeze-Dehydrated Foods." In *Exploration in Future Food-Processing Techniques*, edited by S. A. Goldblith, 54–69. Cambridge, MA: Massachusetts Institute of Technology, 1963.

Kendrick, Douglas B., Leonard D. Heaton, John Boyd Coates, and Elizabeth M. McFetridge. *Blood Program in World War II.* Washington, DC: Office of the Surgeon General, Department of the Army, 1964.

Kurlansky, Mark. *Salt: A World History.* New York: Penguin Books, 2003.

Labuza, Theodore. Interview by the author, May 28, 2013.

———. *Storage Stability and Improvement of Intermediate Moisture Foods: Phase 2.* Houston, TX: Food and Nutrition Office, National Aeronautics and Space Administration, 1974.

Milham, Frederick Heaton. "A Brief History of Shock." *Surgery* 148, no. 5 (2010): 1026–37.

Moss, Michael. "The Hard Sell on Salt." *New York Times*, May 30, 2010, A1.

———. *Salt, Sugar, Fat: How the Food Giants Hooked Us.* New York: Random House, 2013.

Murphy, William P., and William G. Workman. "Serum Hepatitis from Pooled Irradiated Dried Plasma." *Journal of American Medicine* 152, no. 15 (1953): 1421–23.

Murray, Donald M., and Warren D. Siemens. "Applications of Aerospace Technology in Industry. A Technology Transfer Profile: Food Technology." Report prepared for the Technology Utilization Office, National Aeronautics and Space Administration. Cambridge, MA: Abt Associates, Inc., 1971.

National Aeronautics and Space Administration. "The Deterioration of Intermediate Moisture Foods." NASA Tech Brief 71-10332. Manned Spacecraft Center, August 1971.

Paddleford, Clementine. "Made in Natick, Served in Space." *Boston Globe,* August 29, 1965, 25.

Pavey, Robert Louis. *Fabrication of Food Bars Based on Compression and Molding Matrices.* Natick, MA: Food Laboratory, U.S. Army Natick Laboratories 1969.

"Ration D Bars." Hershey Community Archives. Accessed November 28, 2014. http://www.hersheyarchives.org/essay/details.aspx?EssayId=26.

Salwin, Harold. "The Role of Moisture in Deteriorative Reactions of Dehydrated Foods." In *Freeze-Drying of Foods: Proceedings of a Conference,* 58–74. Washington, DC: National Academy of Sciences–National Research Council, 1962.

Smith, Malcolm C., Jr., Rita M. Rapp, Clayton S. Huber, Paul C. Rambaut, and Norman D. Heidelbaugh. *Apollo Experience Report: Food Systems.* Washington, DC: National Aeronautics and Space Administration, 1974.

Smith, Woodruff D. "Complications of the Commonplace: Tea, Sugar, and Imperialism." *Journal of Interdisciplinary History* 23, no. 2 (1992): 259–78.

Strumia, Max M., and John J. McGraw. "Frozen and Dried Plasma for Civil and Military Use." *Journal of American Medicine* 116, no. 21 (1941): 2378–82.

"The Sugar Act of 1937." *Yale Law Journal* 47, no. 6 (1938): 980–93.

Toops, Diane. "Hitting All the Bars." *Food Processing* 66, no. 3 (2005): 37.

Vaughan, William. Interview by the author, May 15, 2013.

Winpenny, Thomas R. "Milton S. Hershey Ventures into Cuban Sugar." *Pennsylvania History* 62, no. 4 (1995): 491–502.

"Without Enzymes, Biological Reaction Essential to Life Takes 2.3 Billion Years: UNC Study." Biochemistry and Biophysics—UNC School of Medicine, November 11, 2008. Accessed September 2, 2013. http://www.med.unc.edu/biochem/news/without-enzyme-biological-reaction-essential-to-life-takes-2-3-billion-years-unc-study.

Worthy, Ward. "Battelle Process Raises Chocolate Melting Point." *Chemical & Engineering News* 66, no. 19 (1988): 6.

Wrolstad, Ronald E. "Functional Properties of Sugars." In *Food Carbohydrate Chemistry,* 77. Hoboken, NJ: Wiley-Blackwell, 2012.

CHAPTER 8. HOW DO YOU WANT THAT CHUNKED AND FORMED RESTRUCTURED STEAK?

American Meat Institute Foundation. *The Science of Meat and Meat Products.* San Francisco: Freeman, 1960.

Armentano, D. T. "The Failure of Antitrust Policy." *The Freeman: Ideas on Liberty,* June 1994: 7.

Armour and Company. *Food for Freedom: Armour and Company's Part in America's All-Out War Effort.* Chicago: Armour and Company, 1942.

Arnould, Richard J. "Changing Patterns of Concentration in American Meat Packing, 1880–1963." *Business History Review* 45, no. 1 (1971): 18–34.

Bettcher, Louis A. Trimming and slicing device. U.S. Patent 25,947, filed for reissue March 2, 1964, and reissued December 14, 1965.

Brand, Charles J. "Some Fertilizer History Connected with World War I." *Agricultural History* 19, no. 2 (1945): 104–13.

Carnes, Richard B. "Meatpacking and Prepared Meats Industry: Above-Average Productivity Gains." *Monthly Labor Review* (April 1984): 37–42.

Cassidy, Elliott. *The Development of Meat, Dairy, Poultry, and Fish Products for the Army.* Washington, DC: Government Printing Office, 1944.

Condon, Howard M. Meat product and method of treating meat. U.S. Patent 2,527,493, filed March 27, 1947, and issued October 24, 1950.

Davies, A. R., and R. J. Board. *The Microbiology of Meat and Poultry.* London: Blackie Academic & Professional, 1998.

Daw, Joseph. *A Sketch of the Early History of the Worshipful Company of Butchers of London.* London: Worshipful Company of Butchers, 1869.

Ercolini, D., F. Russo, E. Torrieri, P. Masi, and F. Villani. "Changes in the Spoilage-Related Microbiota of Beef during Refrigerated Storage under Different Packaging Conditions." *Applied and Environmental Microbiology* 72, no. 7 (2006): 4663–71.

Erisman, Jan Willem, Mark A. Sutton, James Galloway, Zbigniew Klimont, and Wilfried Winiwarter. "How a Century of Ammonia Synthesis Changed the World." *Nature Geoscience* 1 (2008): 636–39.

Farouk, Mustafa. E-mail correspondence with the author, April 2013.

Freidberg, Susanne. *Fresh: A Perishable History.* Cambridge, MA: Belknap Press of Harvard University Press, 2009.

Friedmann, Karen. "Victualling Colonial Boston." *Agricultural History* 47, no. 3 (1973): 189–205.

Gwilliam, Glenn B. Process for manufacturing steak product. U.S. Patent 2,823,127, filed February 24, 1956, and issued February 11, 1958.

Haber, Fritz. "The Synthesis of Ammonia from Its Elements, Nobel Lecture, June 2, 1920." *Resonance* 7, no. 9 (2002): 86–94.

Halper, Emanuel B. *Shopping Center and Store Leases.* Rev. ed. New York: Law Journal Seminars-Press, 1991.

Hawkins, Arthur E., and Jeremy R. Evans. Process for preparing a restructured meat product. U.S. Patent 3,793,466, filed June 11, 1971, and issued February 19, 1974.

Hinnergardt, L. C., R. W. Mandigo, and J. M. Tuomy. "Accelerated Pork Processing: Freeze-Dried Pork Chops." *Journal of Food Science* 38, no. 5 (1973): 831–33.

Huffman, Dale. Interviews by the author, April 2 and 11, 2013.

——. Process for production of a restructured fresh meat product. U.S. Patent 4,210,677, filed January 24, 1978, and issued July 1, 1980.

Hui, Y. H. *Handbook of Meat and Meat Processing.* 2nd ed. Boca Raton, FL: CRC Press, 2012.

——. *Meat Science and Applications.* New York: Marcel Dekker, 2001.

"Iowa Beef Processors, Boxed Beef and a New 'Big Four.'" Wessels Living History Farm. Accessed June 13, 2013. http://www.livinghistoryfarm.org/farminginthe50s/money_17.html.

Jay, James M. *Modern Food Microbiology.* New York: Van Nostrand Reinhold, 1970.

Kerry, J. P., and J. F. Kerry. *Processed Meats: Improving Safety, Nutrition and Quality.* Cambridge, UK: Woodhead Publishing, 2011.

Klont, R. E., L. Brocks, and G. Eikelenboom. "Muscle Fiber Type and Meat Quality." *Meat Science* 49, supplement 1 (1998): S219–29.

Lhuissier, Anne. "Cuts and Classification: The Use of Nomenclatures as a Tool for the Reform of the Meat Trade in France, 1850–1880." *Food and Foodways* 10, no. 4 (2002): 183–208.

Maas, Russell H. Processing meat. U.S. Patent 3,076,713, filed July 3, 1961, and issued February 5, 1963.

MacDonald, James M. "Structural Changes: Location and Plant Operation." In *Consolidation in U.S. Meatpacking,* 12–16. Washington, DC: Economic Research Service, U.S. Department of Agriculture, 2000.

MacDonald, James M., and Michael E. Ollinger. "Technology, Labor Wars, and Producer Dynamics: Explaining Consolidating in Beef-Packing." *American Journal of Agricultural Economics* 87, no. 4 (2005): 1020–33.

Mandigo, Roger. "Fabricated Pork." *Nebraska Swine Report,* January 1, 1972, 6–7.

———. Interview by the author, April 15, 2013.

Mandigo, R. W., and J. F. Campbell. "Cooking, Reheating Restructured Pork Products." *Nebraska Swine Report,* January 1, 1977, 19–20.

Mandigo, Roger W., Louise W. Dalton, and Dennis G. Olson. "Big Chops from Little Pieces." *Nebraska Swine Report,* January 1, 1980, 3–4.

Mandigo, R. W., K. L. Neer, M. S. Chesney, and G. R. Popenhagen. "Restructured Pork: Dollars and Sense." *Nebraska Swine Report,* January 1, 1974, 11–12.

"Military Meat and Dairy Hygiene." *Office of Medical History.* Accessed June 13, 2013. http://history.amedd.army.mil/booksdocs/wwii/vetservicewwii/chapter20.htm.

Moser, Whet. "The Invention of the McRib and Why It Disappears from McDonald's." *Chicago Magazine,* October 25, 2011. Accessed June 13, 2013. http://www.chicagomag.com/Chicago-Magazine/The-312/October-2011/The-Invention-of-the-McRib-and-Why-It-Disappears-from-McDonalds/.

National Academy of Sciences–National Research Council. *Beef for Tomorrow: Proceedings of a Conference.* Washington, DC: National Academy of Sciences–National Research Council, 1960.

Nowak, Dariusz. "Enzymes in Tenderization of Meat—the System of Calpains and Other Systems—a Review." *Polish Journal of Food and Nutrition Sciences* 61, no. 4 (2011): 231–37.

Ofori, Jack Appiah, and Yun-Hwa Peggy Hsieh. "The Use of Blood and Derived Products as Food Additives." In *Food Additives,* edited by Yehia El-Samragy, 229–56. New York: InTech, 2012.

Plumptre, James. *The experienced butcher: shewing the respectability and usefulness of his calling, the religious considerations arising from it, the laws relating to it, and various profitable suggestions for the rightly carrying it on: designed not only for the use of butchers, but also for families and readers in general.* London: Printed for Darton, Harvey, and Darton, 1816.

Sabine, Ernest. "Butchering in Medieval London." *Speculum* (July 1933): 3.

Salant, Abner. Interview by the author, April 25, 2013.

Samat, Maguelonne. *A History of Food.* Oxford: Blackwell Reference, 1993.

Scalzo, Julia. "All a Matter of Taste: The Problem of Victorian and Edwardian Shop Fronts." *Journal of the Society of Architectural Historians* 68, no. 1 (2009): 52–73.

Secrist, John. Interviews by the author, March 26 and April 9, 2013.

Smil, Vaclav. "Eating Meat: Evolution, Patterns, and Consequences." *Population and Development Review* 28, no. 4 (2002): 599–639.

Sobel, Dava. "Making Steak out of Meat Scraps." *Sarasota Herald-Tribune,* January 6, 1980, 60.

Stout, Thomas T., and Murray H. Hawkins. "Implications of Changes in the Methods of Wholesaling Meat Products." *American Journal of Agricultural Economics* 50, no. 3 (1968): 660.

Tinstman, Dale. *Iowa Beef Processors, Inc.: An Entire Industry Revolutionized!* Exton, PA: Newcomen, 1981.

Tischer, Robert, James M. Blair, and Martin Peterson. *Quality and Stability of Canned Meats: A Symposium.* National Academy of Sciences–National Research Council, March 31–April 1, 1953.

Toldrá, Fidel, ed. *Handbook of Meat Processing.* Ames, IA: Wiley-Blackwell, 2010.

———. *Meat Biotechnology.* New York: Springer, 2008.

Tyson Foods, Inc. *Fiscal 2012 Fact Book.* Springdale, AK: Tyson Foods, Inc., 2013.

Walford, Cornelius. *Gilds: Their Origin, Constitution, Objects, and Later History.* New and enl. ed. London: George Redway, 1888.

Walsh, John P. "The Social Context of Technological Change: The Case of the Retail Food Industry." *Sociological Quarterly* 32, no. 3 (1991): 44768.

———. *Supermarkets Transformed: Understanding Organizational and Technological Innovations.* New Brunswick, NJ: Rutgers University Press, 1993.

Wansink, Brian. "Changing Eating Habits on the Home Front: Lost Lessons from World War II Research." *Journal of Public Policy & Marketing* 21, no. 1 (2002): 90–99.

Weightman, Gavin. *The Frozen-Water Trade: A True Story.* New York: Hyperion, 2003.

Wittenberg, J. B., and B. A. Wittenberg. "Myoglobin-Enhanced Oxygen Delivery to Isolated Cardiac Mitochondria." *Journal of Experimental Biology* 210, no. 12 (2007): 2082–90.

CHAPTER 9. A LOAF OF EXTENDED-LIFE BREAD, A HUNK OF PROCESSED CHEESE, AND THOU

Agricultural Research Administration, U.S. Department of Agriculture. *Experimental Compression of Dehydrated Foods.* Washington, DC: Agricultural Research Administration, U.S. Department of Agriculture, 1948.

Araujo, Pedro Soares de, and Anita D. Panek. "The Interaction of *Saccharomyces cerevisiae* Trehalase with Membranes." *Biochimica et Biophysica Acta (BBA)— Biomembranes* 1148, no. 2 (1993): 303–7.

Belderok, B. *Bread-Making Quality of Wheat: A Century of Breeding in Europe.* Dordrecht, Neth.: Kluwer Academic Publishers, 2000.

Bobrow-Strain, Aaron. "Making White Bread by the Bomb's Early Light: Anxiety, Abundance, and Industrial Food Power in the Early Cold War." *Food and Foodways* 19 (2011): 74–97.

Bolat, Irina. "The Importance of Trehalose in Brewing Yeast Survival." *Innovative Romanian Food Biotechnology* 2 (2008): 1–10.

Burrington, Kimberlee J. "Understanding Process Cheeses." *Food Product Design,* February 1, 2000.

Caputo, Ivana, Marilena Lepretti, Stefania Martucciello, and Carla Esposito. "Enzymatic Strategies to Detoxify Gluten: Implications for Celiac Disease." *Enzyme Research,* 2010 (2010): 1–9.

Cauvain, Stanley P., and Linda S. Young. *Baked Products: Science, Technology and Practice.* Oxford: Blackwell, 2006.

———. *Technology of Breadmaking.* 2nd ed. New York: Springer, 2007.

Chinachoti, Pavinee. *Bread Staling.* Boca Raton, FL: CRC Press, 2001.

———. E-mail correspondence with the author, May 2014.

Cole, Martin. Interviews by the author, April 2 and May 12, 2014.

Conn, James Fred. "Fungal Enzyme Preparations as Alpha-Amylase Supplements in Baking." Master's thesis, Department of Milling Industry, Kansas State College, 1949.

Cowgill, George R. "Some Food Problems in War Time." *American Scientist* 31, no. 2 (1943): 142–50.

Cunha, Clarissa R., and Walkiria H. Viotto. "Casein Peptization, Functional Properties, and Sensory Acceptance of Processed Cheese Spreads Made with Different Emulsifying Salts." *Journal of Food Science* 75, no. 1 (2010): C113–20.

Day, L., M. A. Augustin, I. L. Batey, and C. W. Wrigley. "Wheat-Gluten Uses and Industry Needs." *Trends in Food Science & Technology* 17 (2006): 82–90.

Economou, Michael, and Georgios Pappas. "New Global Map of Crohn's Disease: Genetic, Environmental, and Socioeconomic Correlations." *Inflammatory Bowel Diseases* 14, no. 5 (2008): 709–20.

Eliasson, Ann-Charlotte, and Kare Larsson. *Cereals in Breadmaking: A Molecular Colloidal Approach.* New York: Marcel Dekker, 1993.

Erba, Eric M., and Andrew M. Novakovic. *The Evolution of Milk Pricing and Government Intervention in Dairy Markets.* Ithaca, NY: Cornell Program on Dairy Markets and Policy, 1995.

Fernandes, Pedro. "Enzymes in Food Processing: A Condensed Overview on Strategies for Better Biocatalysts." *Enzyme Research* 2010 (2010): 1–19.

Fox, Patrick. E-mail correspondence with the author, April 2014.

———. *Fundamentals of Cheese Science.* Gaithersburg, MD: Aspen Publishers, 2000.

Gates, Robert Leroy. "Preparation of Amylase Active Concentrates from Mold Bran." Master's thesis, Department of Milling Industry, Kansas State College, 1947.

Gilpin, Kenneth N. "Nabisco in Accord to Be Purchased by Philip Morris." *New York Times,* June 26, 2000.

Goesaert, Hans, Louise Slade, Harry Levine, and Jan A. Delcour. "Amylases and Bread Firming—an Integrated View." *Journal of Cereal Science* 50 (2009): 345–52.

Gray, J. A., and J. N. Bemiller. "Bread Staling: Molecular Basis and Control." *Comprehensive Reviews in Food Science and Food Safety* 2, no. 1 (2003): 1–21.

Gupta, Rani, Paresh Gigras, Harapriya Mohapatra, Vineet Kumar Goswami, and Bhavna Chauhan. "Microbial α-Amylases: A Biotechnological Perspective." *Process Biochemistry* 38, no. 11 (2003): 1599–616.

Hallberg, Linnea M., and Pavinee Chinachota. "A Fresh Perspective on Staling: The Significance of Starch Crystallization on the Firming of Bread." *Journal of Food Science* 67, no. 3 (2002): 1092–96.

Herz, Matthew L. *Proceedings of the Natick Science Symposium (3rd) Held in Natick, Massachusetts on 5–6 June 1990.* Fort Belvoir, VA: Defense Technical Information Center, 1990.

Hillson, S. W. "Diet and Dental Disease." *World Archaeology* 11, no. 2 (1979): 147–62.

Ingraham, John L. *March of the Microbes: Sighting the Unseen.* Cambridge, MA: Belknap Press Imprint, 2012.

Jackel, S. S., A. S. Schultz, and W. E. Schaeder. "Susceptibility of the Starch in Fresh and Stale Bread to Enzymatic Digestion." *Science* 118 (1953): 18–19.

Kang, J. Y., A. H. Y. Kang, A. Green, K. A. Gwee, and K. Y. Ho. "Systematic Review: Worldwide Variation in the Frequency of Coeliac Disease and Changes over Time." *Alimentary Pharmacology & Therapeutics* 38, no. 3 (2013): 226–45.

Kasapis, Stefan. "Recent Advances and Future Challenges in the Explanation and Exploitation of the Network Glass Transition of High Sugar/Biopolymer Mixtures." *Critical Reviews in Food Science and Nutrition* 48, no. 2 (2008): 185–203.

Kohajdová, Zlatica, Jolana Karovičová, and Štefan Schmidt. "Significance of Emulsifiers and Hydrocolloids in Bakery Industry." *Acta Chimica Slovaca* 2, no. 1 (2009): 46–61.

Labuza, T. P., and C. R. Hyman. "Moisture Migration and Control in Multi-Domain Foods." *Trends in Food Science & Technology* 9, no. 2 (1998): 47–55.

Lester, Diane R. "Gluten Measurement and Its Relationship to Food Toxicity for Celiac Disease Patients." *Plant Methods* 4 (2008): 4–26.

Levine, Harry, and Louise Slade. "Glass Transitions in Food." In *Physical Chemistry of Foods,* edited by Henry G. Schwartzberg and Richard W. Hartel, 83–221. New York: Marcel Dekker, Inc., 1992.

Megahed, Mohamed G. "Preparation of Sucrose Fatty Acid Esters as Food Emulsifiers and Evaluation of Their Surface Active and Emulsification Properties." *Grasas y Aceites* 50, no. 4 (1999): 280–82.

McHarry, Samuel. *The practical distiller, or, An introduction to making whiskey, gin, brandy, spirits, &c. &c. of better quality and in larger quantities than produced by the present mode of distilling, from the produce of the United States* . . . Harrisburgh, PA: John Wyeth, 1809.

Nanninga, Nanne. "Did van Leeuwenhoek Observe Yeast Cells in 1680?" *Small Things Considered*, April 8, 2010. http://schaechter.asmblog.org/schaechter/2010/04/did -van-leeuwenhoek-observe-yeast-cells-in-1680.html.

Oleksyk, Lauren. Interview by the author, April 17, 2014.

Orthoefer, Frank. "Applications of Emulsifiers in Baked Foods." In *Food Emulsifiers and Their Applications*, 2nd ed., edited by Gerard L. Hasenhuettl, 267–84. New York: Springer, 2008.

Otterstedt, Karin, Christer Larsson, Roslyn M. Bill, Anders Ståhlberg, Eckhard Boles, Stefan Hohmann, and Lena Gustafsson. "Switching the Mode of Metabolism in the Yeast *Saccharomyces cerevisiae*." *EMBO Reports* 5, no. 5 (2004): 532–37.

"Our Bread-Eating Army in France." *Army and Navy Register*, January 4, 1919, 44–45.

Pain, Stephanie. "Why the Pharaohs Never Smiled: Life in Ancient Egypt Was Very Civilised—Until You Needed a Dentist. Stephanie Pain Gets to the Root of the Matter." *New Scientist*, July 2, 2005, 36–40.

Porta, Raffaele, Ashok Pandey, and Cristina M. Rosell. "Enzymes as Additives or Processing Aids in Food Biotechnology." *Enzyme Research* 2010 (2010): 1–2.

Radovich, John M. "Mass Transfer Effects in Fermentations Using Immobilized Whole Cells." *Enzyme and Microbial Technology* 7, no. 1 (1985): 2–10.

Red Star Yeast & Products Co. v. Commissioner of Internal Revenue, Docket No. 48691, 25 T.C. 321 (1955).

Reed, Gerald. "Milling and Baking." In *Enzymes in Food Processing*, 221–55. New York: Academic Press, 1966.

Rinaldi, Maurizio, Roberto Perricone, Miri Blank, Carlo Perricone, and Yehuda Shoenfeld. "Anti-*Saccharomyces cerevisiae* Autoantibodies in Autoimmune Diseases: From Bread Baking to Autoimmunity." *Clinical Reviews in Allergy & Immunology* 45, no. 2 (2013): 152–61.

Ross, William F., and Charles F. Romanus. *The Quartermaster Corps: Operations in the War against Germany*. U.S. Army in World War II. 1965. Reprint, Washington, DC: United States Army, 1991.

Samuel, D. "Investigation of Ancient Egyptian Baking and Brewing Methods by Correlative Microscopy." *Science* 273, no. 5274 (1996): 488–90.

Shadbolt, Peter. "Tomb of Ancient Egypt's Beer Maker to Gods of the Dead Discovered." CNN, January 20, 2014. Accessed April 10, 2014. http://www.cnn.com/2014/01/20/world/meast/egypt-ancient-beer-brewer-tomb/.

Shellenberger, J. A. "The History of the Department of Milling Industry, 1910–1966." Manhattan: Kansas State University, 1970.

Slade, Louise. E-mail correspondence with the author, May 2014.

Stone, Irwin. Retarding the staling of bakery products. U.S. Patent 2615810A, filed March 4, 1948, and issued October 28, 1952.

Sutton, K. H., N. G. Larsen, M. P. Morgenstern, M. Ross, L. D. Simmons, and A. J. Wilson. "Differing Effects of Mechanical Dough Development and Sheeting Development Methods on Aggregated Glutenin Proteins." *Cereal Chemistry* 80, no. 6 (2003): 707–11.

Tamime, A. Y. *Processed Cheese and Analogues.* Oxford: Wiley-Blackwell, 2011.

Teal, A. R., and P. E. O. Wymer. *Enzymes and Their Role in Biotechnology.* London: Biochemical Society, 1991.

Uthayakumaran, S., M. Newberry, M. Keentok, F. L. Stoddard, and F. Bekes. "Basic Rheology of Bread Dough with Modified Protein Content and Glutenin-to-Gliadin Ratios." *Cereal Chemistry* 77, no. 6 (2000): 744–49.

Wade, Marcia A. "Cheese Powder—the Ingredient Chameleon." *Prepared Foods,* January 1, 2004.

Welch, R. W., and P. C. Mitchell. "Food Processing: A Century of Change." *British Medical Bulletin* 56, no. 1 (2000): 1–17.

Wiemken, Andres. "Trehalose in Yeast, Stress Protectant Rather Than Reserve Carbohydrate." *Antonie van Leeuwenhoek* 58, no. 3 (1990): 209–17.

Wieser, Herbert. "Chemistry of Gluten Proteins." *Food Microbiology* 24, no. 2 (2007): 115–19.

Wieser, Herbert, and Peter Koehler. "The Biochemical Basis of Celiac Disease." *Cereal Chemistry* 85, no. 1 (2008): 1–13.

Wilford, John Noble. "In Ancient Egypt, the Beer of Kings Was a Sophisticated Brew." *New York Times,* July 26, 1996.

Zheng, H., M. P. Morgenstern, O. H. Campanella, and N. G. Larsen. "Rheological Properties of Dough during Mechanical Dough Development." *Journal of Cereal Science* 32, no. 3 (2000): 293–306.

CHAPTER 10. PLASTIC PACKAGING REMODELS THE PLANET

American Chemical Society National Historic Chemical Landmarks. "Foundations of Polymer Science: Herman Mark and the Polymer Research Institute." Accessed November 15, 2014. http://www.acs.org/content/acs/en/education/whatischemis try/landmarks/polymerresearchinstitute.html.

Azeredo, Henriette. "Nanocomposites for Food Packaging Applications." *Food Research International* 42, no. 9 (2009): 1240–53.

Aznar, M., M. Canellas, and E. Gaspar. "Migration from Food Packaging Laminates Based on Polyurethane." *Italian Journal of Food Science* 23, SI (2011): 95–98.

Bang, Du Yeon, Hyung Sik Kim, Bu Young Jung, Min Ji Kim, Minji Kyung, Byung Mu Lee, Youngkwan Lee, et al. "Human Risk Assessment of Endocrine-Disrupting Chemicals Derived from Plastic Food Containers." *Comprehensive Reviews in Food Science and Food Safety* 11, no. 5 (2012): 453–70.

Bhunia, Kanishka, Shyam S. Sablani, Juming Tang, and Barbara Rasco. "Migration of Chemical Compounds from Packaging Polymers during Microwave, Conventional Heat Treatment, and Storage." *Comprehensive Reviews in Food Science and Food Safety* 12, no. 5 (2013): 523–45.

Blair, Etcyl. "History of Chemistry in the Dow Chemical Company." Speech given at the Central Regional Meeting, American Chemical Society, Midland, Michigan, May 18, 2006.

Blewett, J. P., and J. H. Rubel. "Video Delay Lines." *Proceedings of the IRE* 35, no. 12 (1947): 1580–84.

Boyer, Raymond F. "Herman Mark and the Plastics Industry." *Journal of Polymer Science Part C: Polymer Symposia* 12, no. 1 (1966): 111–18.

———. Interview by James J. Bohning at Michigan Molecular Institute, Midland, Michigan, January 14 and August 19, 1986. Oral history transcript #0015, Chemical Heritage Foundation, Philadelphia.

———. Vinylidene chloride compositions stable to light. U.S. Patent 2,429,155A, filed May 4, 1945, and issued October 14, 1947.

Brody, Aaron. Interview by the author, June 11, 2014.

Brody, Aaron L., and Eugene R. Strupinsky. *Active Packaging for Food Applications*. Lancaster, PA: Technomic Publishing, 2001.

Cao, Xu-Liang. "Phthalate Esters in Foods: Sources, Occurrence, and Analytical Methods." *Comprehensive Reviews in Food Science and Food Safety* 9, no. 1 (2010): 21–43.

Carnegie Institution. "Hydrocarbons in the Deep Earth?" *ScienceDaily,* July 27, 2009. Accessed May 16, 2014. http://www.sciencedaily.com/releases/2009/07/090726150843.htm.

Clark, J. Peter. "Retort Pouch Foods." In *Case Studies in Food Engineering: Learning from Experience,* 91–101. New York: Springer, 2009.

Cochrane, Rexmond C. "World War II Research (1941–1945)." In *Measures for Progress: A History of the National Bureau of Standards,* 365–426. Washington, DC: National Institute of Standards and Technology, 1966.

Connan, J. "Use and Trade of Bitumen in Antiquity and Prehistory: Molecular Archaeology Reveals Secrets of Past Civilizations." *Philosophical Transactions of the Royal Society B: Biological Sciences* 354, no. 1379 (1999): 33–50.

Craven, W. F., and J. L. Cate. "Allocation and Distribution of Aircraft." In *The Army Air Forces in World War II, Part VI: Men and Planes,* edited by Wesley Frank Craven and James Lea Gate. Washington, DC: Government Printing Office, 1983.

Darsch, Gerald, and Stephen Moody. "The Packaged Military Meal." In *Meals in Science and Practice: Interdisciplinary Research and Business,* edited by H. L. Meiselman, 297–342. Cambridge, UK: Woodhead Publishing, 2009.

Duncan, Timothy V. "Applications of Nanotechnology in Food Packaging and Food Safety: Barrier Materials, Antimicrobials and Sensors." *Journal of Colloid and Interface Science* 363, no. 1 (2011): 1–24.

Dunn, Thomas J., and Amy W. Sherrill. *Light Barrier for Non-Foil Packaging.* Natick, MA: Defense Technical Information Center, 2010.

Dunn, Thomas. Interview by the author, June 9, 2014.

"DuPont: Powder, Paint and Perambulators." *New York Times,* April 6, 1919.

Egloff, Gustav. "Peacetime Values from a War Technology." *Science,* January 29, 1943, 2509.

Elliott, Kevin C., and David C. Volz. "Addressing Conflicts of Interest in Nanotechnology Oversight: Lessons Learned from Drug and Pesticide Safety Testing." *Journal of Nanoparticle Research* 14, no. 1 (2012): 1–5.

Factor-Litvak P., B. Insel, A. M. Calafat, X. Liu, F. Perera, V. A. Rauh, and R. M. Whyatt. "Persistent Associations between Maternal Prenatal Exposure to Phthalates on Child IQ at Age 7 Years." *PLoS One,* December 10, 2014.

Fasano, Evelina, Francisco Bono-Blay, Teresa Cirillo, Paolo Montuori, and Silvia Lacorte. "Migration of Phthalates, Alkylphenols, Bisphenol A and Di(2-ethylhexyl) adipate from Food Packaging." *Food Control* 27, no. 1 (2012): 132–38.

Feilchenfeld, Hans. "Bond Length and Bond Energy in Hydrocarbons." *Journal of Physical Chemistry* 61, no. 9 (1957): 1133–35.

Field, Hugh W. "New Products of the Petroleum Industry." *Journal of The Franklin Institute* 243, no. 2 (1947): 95–116.

Forbes, R. J. "Petroleum and Bitumen in Antiquity." *Ambix* 2, no. 2 (1938): 68–92.

Freemantle, Michael. "What's That Stuff? Asphalt." *Chemical & Engineering News* 77, no. 44 (1999): 81.

Froio, Danielle, Jeanne Lucciarini, Christopher Thellen, and Jo Ann Ratto. *Nanocomposites Research for Combat Ration Packaging.* Fort Belvoir, VA: Defense Technical Information Center, 2004.

Froio, Danielle, Jeanne Lucciarini, Christopher Thellen, Jo Ann Ratto, and Elizabeth Culhane. *Developments in High Barrier Non-Foil Packaging Structures for Military Rations.* Fort Belvoir, VA: Defense Technical Information Center, 2005.

Han, Jung H. *Innovations in Food Packaging.* San Diego, CA: Elsevier Academic, 2005.

Hanson, Luther. Interview by the author, May 23, 2014.

Hartung, Thomas. "A Toxicology for the 21st Century—Mapping the Road Ahead." *Toxicological Sciences* 109, no. 1 (2009): 18–23.

Hauser, R., J. D. Meeker, N. P. Singh, M. J. Silva, L. Ryan, S. Duty, and A. M. Calafat. "DNA Damage in Human Sperm Is Related to Urinary Levels of Phthalate Monoester and Oxidative Metabolites." *Human Reproduction* 22, no. 3 (2006): 688–95.

Hounshell, David A., and John K. Smith. *Science and Corporate Strategy: Du Pont R&D, 1902–1980.* Cambridge: Cambridge University Press, 1988.

Hunt, Morton. "Polymers Everywhere, Parts I and II." *New Yorker,* September 13 and 20, 1958.

Karel, Marcus, and Gerald Wogan. "Migration of Substances from Flexible Containers for Heat-Processed Foods." Cambridge, MA: Division of Sponsored Research, Massachusetts Institute of Technology, 1962.

King, Gilbert. "Fritz Haber's Experiments in Life and Death." *Smithsonian Magazine,* June 6, 2012. Accessed November 15, 2014. http://www.smithsonianmag.com/history/fritz-habers-experiments-in-life-and-death-114161301/?no-ist.

Kirwan, Mark J. *Food and Beverage Packaging Technology.* 2nd ed. Ames, IA: Wiley, 2011.

Kunzmann, Andrea, Britta Andersson, Tina Thurnherr, Harald Krug, Annika Scheynius, and Bengt Fadeel. "Toxicology of Engineered Nanomaterials: Focus on Biocompatibility, Biodistribution and Biodegradation." *Biochimica et Biophysica Acta* 1810 (2011): 361–73.

Lampi, Rauno A. "Flexible Packaging for Thermoprocessed Foods." In *Advances in Food Research,* edited by E. M. Mrak, C. O. Chichester, and G. F. Stewart, 305–428. New York: Academic Press, 1977.

———. Interview by the author, June 3, 2014.

Lucciarini, Jeanne M., Jo Ann Ratto, Byron E. Koene, and Bert Powell. "Nanocomposites Study of Ethylene Co-Vinyl Alcohol and Montmorillonite Clay." *Antec* 2 (2002): 1514–18.

Maffini, Maricel V., Heather M. Alger, Erik D. Olson, and Thomas G. Neltner. "Looking Back to Look Forward: A Review of FDA's Food Additives Safety Assessment and Recommendations for Modernizing Its Program." *Comprehensive Reviews in Food Science and Food Safety* 12, no. 4 (2013): 439–53.

Mark, Herman. Interview by James J. Bohning and Jeffrey L. Sturchio at Polytechnic University, Brooklyn, New York, February 3, March 17, and June 20, 1986. Oral history transcript #0030, Chemical Heritage Foundation, Philadelphia.

Mayerson, Philip. "Pitch (πίσσα) for Egyptian Winejars an Imported Commodity." *Zeitschrift für Papyrologie und Epigraphik* 147 (2004): 201–4.

Miller, Margaret A., Weida Tong, Xiaohui Fan, and William Slikker Jr. "2012 Global Summit on Regulatory Science (GSRS-2012)—Modernizing Toxicology." *Toxicological Sciences* 13, no. 1 (2013): 9–12.

Morawetz, Herbert. *Herman Francis Mark 1895–1992.* Washington, DC: National Academies Press, 1995.

Nagarajan, Ramaswamy. Interview with the author, May 27, 2014.

Nowak, Peter. *Sex, Bombs, and Burgers: How War, Pornography, and Fast Food Have Shaped Modern Technology.* Guilford, CT: Lyons Press, 2011.

O'Conner, John J. *Polytechnic Institute of Brooklyn: An Account of the Educational Purposes and Development of the Institute during Its First Century.* Brooklyn, NY: Polytechnic Institute of Brooklyn, 1955.

Ostkr, Gerald. "Research on the Photochemistry of High Polymers at the Polytechnic Institute of Brooklyn." *Journal of Polymer Science Part C: Polymer Symposia* 12, no. 1 (1966): 63–69.

Ozaki, Asako, Yukihiko Yamaguchi, Akiyoshi Okamoto, and Nobuko Kawai. "Determination of Alkylphenols, Bisphenol A, Benzophenone and Phthalates in Containers of Baby Food, and Migration into Food Simulants." *Journal of the Food Hygienic Society of Japan (Shokuhin Eiseigaku Zasshi)* 43, no. 4 (2002): 260–66.

Panessa-Warren, Barbara J., John B. Warren, Mathew M. Maye, and Wynne Schiffer. "Nanoparticle Interactions with Living Systems: In Vivo and In Vitro Biocompatibility." In *Nanoparticles and Nanodevices in Biological Applications: The INFN Lectures,* edited by Stefano Bellucci, 1:1–46. Berlin: Springer Science & Business Media, 2009.

Parkinson, Caroline. "Packaging for Protection." *Science News-Letter,* October 21, 1944, 266–67.

Poole, Charles P., Jr., and Frank J. Owens. *Introduction to Nanotechnology.* Hoboken, NJ: John Wiley & Sons, 2003.

Ratto, Jo Ann. Interview by the author, July 10, 2014.

Ratto, Jo Ann, Jeanne Lucciarini, Christopher Thellen, Danielle Froio, and Nandika A. Souza. *The Reduction of Solid Waste Associated with Military Ration Packaging.* Fort Belvoir, VA: Defense Technical Information Center, 2006.

"Raymond F. Boyer." In *Memorial Tributes: National Academy of Engineering,* 25–27. Washington, DC: National Academies Press, 1994.

Robertson, Gordon L. E-mail correspondence with the author, June 2014.

———. *Food Packaging: Principles and Practice.* 3rd ed. Boca Raton, FL: Taylor & Francis/CRC Press, 2013.

Rubens, Louis C. Interview by James J. Bohning at Midland, Michigan, August 19, 1986. Oral history transcript #0048, Chemical Heritage Foundation, Philadelphia.

Rubinate, Frank J. "Flexible Containers for Heat-Processed Foods." Proceedings of the Conference on Flexible Packaging of Military Items. Chicago: National Academy of Sciences/Quartermaster Food and Container Institute for the Armed Forces, 1960.

Rudel, Ruthann A., Janet M. Gray, Connie L. Engel, Teresa W. Rawsthorne, Robin E. Dodson, Janet M. Ackerman, Jeanne Rizzo, Janet L. Nudelman, and Julia Green Brody. "Food Packaging and Bisphenol A and Bis(2-Ethyhexyl) Phthalate Exposure: Findings from a Dietary Intervention." *Environmental Health Perspectives* 119, no. 7 (2011): 914–20.

"Saran Wrap, Marking 40 Years in Use, Began as Lab Byproduct." *Toledo Blade,* January 25, 1994, 19.

Schirmer, Sarah. "Nanocomposites for Military Food Packaging Applications." Presentation at the 2009 Symposium on Nanomaterials for Flexible Packaging, Technical Association of the Pulp and Paper Industry, Columbus, OH, April 28, 2009.

Smith, Andrew F., ed. "Plastic Covering." In *The Oxford Companion to American Food and Drink,* 465. New York: Oxford University Press, 2007.

Smith, John Kenley. Interview by the author, June 13, 2014.

———. "World War II and the Transformation of the American Chemical Industry." In *Science, Technology and the Military,* edited by E. Mendelsohn, M. R. Smith, and P. Weingart, 307–22. Dordrecht, Neth.: Kluwer Academic Publishers, 1988.

Sorrentino, A., G. Gorrasi, and V. Vittoria. "Potential Perspectives of Bio-Nanocomposites for Food Packaging Applications." *Trends in Food Science & Technology* 18, no. 2 (2007): 84–95.

Stark, Anne M. "Hydrocarbons in the Deep Earth." April 14, 2011. Accessed May 18, 2014. https://www.llnl.gov/news/newsreleases/2011/Apr/NR-11-04-04.html.

Szczeblowski, J. W., and F. J. Rubinate, "Integrity of Food Packages," *Modern Packaging,* June 1965.

Thellen, Christopher, Caitlin Orroth, and JoAnn Ratto. *Thermal Analysis of Nanocomposites: An Overview of Polymer/Montmorillonite Layered Silicate Systems.* Fort Belvoir, VA: Defense Technical Information Center, 2004.

Treuel, Lennart, Xiue Jiang, and Gerd Ulrich Nienhaus. "New Views on Cellular Uptake and Trafficking of Manufactured Nanoparticles." *Journal of the Royal Society Interface* 10, no. 82 (2013): 20120939.

Uddin, Faheem. "Clays, Nanoclays, and Montmorillonite Minerals." *Metallurgical and Materials Transactions* 39, no. 12 (2008): 2804–14.

U.S. Army. *Restricted Research and Development Program.* Philadelphia: Office of the Quartermaster General, Military Planning Division, Research and Development Branch, 1947.

Vandenberg, L. N., T. Colborn, T. B. Hayes, J. J. Heindel, D. R. Jacobs, D. H. Lee, J. P. Myers, et al. "Regulatory Decisions on Endocrine Disrupting Chemicals Should Be Based on the Principles of Endocrinology." *Reproductive Toxicology* 38C (2013): 1–15.

Venable, Charles S., Henry B. McClure, and Jeremy C. Jenks. "Chemical Forum." *Analysts Journal* 7, no. 2 (1951): 117–29.

"War Weapons Canned: Cosmoline Replaced by Plastic Coating, Steel Containers." *New York Times,* November 4, 1945, E9.

Wessling, Richard. E-mail correspondence with the author, June 2014.

Yam, Kit L., ed. *The Wiley Encyclopedia of Packaging Technology.* Malden, MA: Wiley, 2010.

Zimm, Bruno H. Interview by James J. Bohning at Anaheim, California, September 9, 1986. Oral history transcript #0055, Chemical Heritage Foundation, Philadelphia.

CHAPTER 11. LATE-NIGHT MUNCHIES? BREAK OUT THE THREE-YEAR-OLD PIZZA AND MONTHS-OLD GUACAMOLE

Balasubramanian, V. M., Daniel Farkas, and Evan J. Turek. "Preserving Foods through High-Pressure Processing." *Food Technology* 62, no. 11 (2008): 32–38.

Barba, Francisco J., María J. Esteve, and Ana Frígola. "High Pressure Treatment Effect on Physicochemical and Nutritional Properties of Fluid Foods during Storage: A Review." *Comprehensive Reviews in Food Science and Food Safety* 11, no. 3 (2012): 307–22.

Barbosa-Cánovas, Gustavo V., Anthony J. Fontana, Jr.; Shelly J. Schmidt, and Theodore P. Labuza, eds. *Water Activity in Foods: Fundamentals and Applications.* Ames, IA: IFT Press/Blackwell Publishing, 2007.

Barbosa-Cánovas, Gustavo V., Maria S. Tapia, and M. Pilar Cano. *Novel Food Processing Technologies.* Boca Raton, FL: CRC Press, 2004.

Bidlas, Eva, and Ronald J. W. Lambert. "Quantification of Hurdles: Predicting the Combination of Effects—Interaction vs. Non-Interaction." *International Journal of Food Microbiology* 128 (2008): 78–88.

Brown, K. L. "Control of Bacterial Spores." *British Medical Bulletin* 56, no. 1 (2000): 158–71.

Cole, Martin. Interviews by the author, April 2 and May 12, 2014.

Doona, Christopher J., and Florence E. Feeherry. *High Pressure Processing of Foods.* Hoboken, NJ: John Wiley & Sons, 2007.

Dunne, C. Patrick. Interviews by the author, March 24 and July 15, 2014.

Ennen, Steve. "High-Pressure Pioneers Ignite Fresh Approach. (Avomex Foods Use High Pressure Food Processing.)" *Food Processing,* January 1, 2001, 16.

Farkas, Daniel. Interviews by the author, March 17 and March 28, 2014.

Farkas, Daniel F., and Dallas G. Hoover. "High Pressure Processing." *Journal of Food Science* 65 (2000): 47–64.

Hemley, Russell J. "Effects of High Pressure on Molecules." *Annual Review of Physical Chemistry* 51 (2000): 763–800.

Hesseltine, C. W. "Dorothy I. Fennell." *Mycologia* 71, no. 5 (1979): 889–91.

Hite, Bert Holmes. *The Effect of Pressure in the Preservation of Milk.* West Virginia Agricultural Experiment Station Bulletin 58. Morgantown: West Virginia Agricultural Experiment Station, 1899.

Holley, Richard A., and Dhaval Patel. "Improvement in Shelf-Life and Safety of Perishable Foods by Plant Essential Oils and Smoke Antimicrobials." *Food Microbiology* 22, no. 4 (2005): 273–92.

Kotula, Kathryn. E-mail correspondence with the author, August 2014.

Kurlansky, Mark. *Salt: A World History.* New York: Walker & Company, 2002.

Leistner, Lothar. "Basic Aspects of Food Preservation by Hurdle Technology." *International Journal of Food Microbiology* 55, no. 1–3 (2000): 181–86.

———. E-mail correspondence with the author, September 2011.

———. "Further Developments in the Utilization of Hurdle Technology for Food Preservation." *Journal of Food Engineering* 22, no. 1–4 (1994): 421–32.

Leistner, Lothar, and Leon G. M. Gorris. "Food Preservation by Hurdle Technology." *Trends in Food Science & Technology* 6, no. 2 (1995): 41–46.

Marler, Bill. "Another Lesson Learned the Hard Way: Odwalla *E. coli* Outbreak 1996." *Marler Blog,* January 23, 2013. Accessed March 23, 2014. http://www.marlerblog .com/legal-cases/another-lesson-learned-the-hard-way-odwalla-e-coli-outbreak -1996/.

Oleksyk, Lauren. Interview by the author, April 17, 2014.

"Pressure-Assisted Sterilization Accepted by FDA." *Food Processing,* March 6, 2009. Accessed March 24, 2014. http://www.foodprocessing.com/articles/2009/032/.

Richardson, Michelle. Interview by the author, July 10, 2014.

Roos, Yrjö H. *Phase Transitions in Foods.* San Diego, CA: Academic Press, 1995.

Sizer, Charles. Interview by the author, March 28, 2014.

Ting, Edmund. Interview by the author, March 26, 2014.

U.S. Food and Drug Administration. "Final Rule: Hazard Analysis and Critical Control Point (HACCP); Procedures for the Safe and Sanitary Processing and Importing of Juice." 66 Fed. Reg. (Jan. 19, 2001): 6138202.

———. "Kinetics of Microbial Inactivation for Alternative Food Processing Technologies." Accessed March 14, 2014. http://www.fda.gov/food/foodscienceresearch/ safepracticesforfoodprocesses/ucm101456.htm.

CHAPTER 12. SUPERMARKET TOUR

Bauman, Howard E., and Robert P. Wooden. "Food Safety Management Systems." *Proceedings of the 43rd Reciprocal Meat Conference, American Meat Science Association, June 1990, Mississippi State University.*

Brody, Aaron. Interview by the author, June 11, 2014.

Buchanan, Nicholas. "The Atomic Meal: The Cold War and Irradiated Foods, 1945–1963." *History and Technology: An International Journal* 21, no. 2 (2005): 221–49.

"Chiquita Brands International to Acquire Fresh Express," financial release, Chiquita Brands International, Inc., February 23, 2005.

"Florida Foods, Inc., Plans 5,500-lb. Powdered Orange Juice Production Per Day." *Billboard*, January 12, 1946, 84.

Holsten, D., M. Sugii, and F. Steward. "Direct and Indirect Effects of Radiation on Plant Cells: Their Relation to Growth and Growth Induction." *Nature* 208 (1965): 850.

Karp, Aaron. "FAA: US Commercial Aircraft Fleet Shrank in 2011." *Air Transport World*, March 12, 2012. Accessed October 26, 2014. http://atwonline.com/aircraft-amp-engines/faa-us-commercial-aircraft-fleet-shrank-2011.

Kent, George. "Two Practical Men Revolutionize the Processing of Rice." *Washington Post*, January 16, 1944, B6.

Lyons, Richard. "Drug Agency Officials Caution on Safety of Irradiated Meats." *New York Times*, July 31, 1968, 52.

Mead, Margaret. "The Factor of Food Habits." In "Nutrition and Food Supply: The War and After," *Annals of the American Academy of Political and Social Science* 225 (1943): 136–41.

Meiselman, Herbert L., and Howard G. Schutz. *History of Food Acceptance Research in the US Army.* Lincoln, NE: U.S. Army Research, U.S. Department of Defense, 2003.

Morris, Charles E. "75 Years of Food Frontiers." *Food Engineering* 75, no. 9 (2003): 54–63.

"National Nutrition Conference for Defense." *Journal of the American Medical Association* 116, no. 23 (1941): 2598.

Radiation Sterilization of Food: Hearing Before the Subcommittee on Research and Development of the Joint Committee on Atomic Energy. 84th Cong., May 9, 1955.

Ross-Nazzal, Jennifer. "From Farm to Fork: How Space Food Standards Impacted the Food Industry and Changed Food Safety Standards." In *Societal Impact of Spaceflight*, edited by Steven J. Dick and Roger D. Launius, 219–36. Washington, DC: NASA, Office of External Relations, History Division, 2007.

"Scientific Proceedings, Forty-Seventh General Meeting of the Society of American Bacteriologists." *Journal of Bacteriology* 54, no. 1 (1947): 30.

Spiller, James. "Radiant Cuisine: The Commercial Fate of Food Irradiation in the United States." *Technology and Culture* 45, no. 4 (2004): 740–63.

Wansink, Brian. "Changing Eating Habits on the Home Front: Lost Lessons from World War II Research." *Journal of Public Policy & Marketing* 21, no. 1 (2002): 90–99.

CHAPTER 13. COMING UP NEXT FROM THE HOUSE OF GI JOE

Armstrong, Robert E. *Bio-Inspired Innovation and National Security.* Washington, DC: Center for Technology and National Security Policy, National Defense University Press, 2010.

Carrier Corporation, Carrier Transicold Container. "Turn to the Experts Refrigeration Boot Camp." Accessed November 21, 2013. files.carrier.com/container-refrigeration/en/worldwide/contentimages/CL_10_12.pdf.

Farrell, Stephen, and Elisabeth Bumiller. "No Shortcuts When Military Moves a War." *New York Times,* March 31, 2010.

Fitzgerald, Warren B., Oliver J. A. Howitt, Inga J. Smith, and Anthony Hume. "Energy Use of Integral Refrigerated Containers in Maritime Transportation." *Energy Policy* 39, no. 4 (2011): 1885–96.

Given, Zack, and Chad Haering. *Performance Evaluation of Two Prototype Beverage Chillers in a Field Environment.* Natick, MA: U.S. Army Natick Soldier Research, Development and Engineering Center, 2012.

Gourley, Scott R. "Shipping Out ISO-Based Deployment Systems." Defense Media Network, June 18, 2010. Accessed November 22, 2013. http://www.defensemedia network.com/stories/shipping-out-ISO-based-deployment-systems/.

Intralytix. Press releases, 2008–13.

Izenson, M., W. Chen, C. W. Haering, J. Sung, and D. Pickard. *Convective Evaporation through Water-Permeable Membranes for Rapid Beverage Chilling.* Natick, MA: U.S. Army Natick Soldier Research, Development and Engineering Center, 2008.

Kalinichev, A. G., and J. D. Bass. "Hydrogen Bonding in Supercritical Water. 2. Computer Simulations." *Journal of Physical Chemistry* 101, no. 50 (1997): 9720–27.

Kaushik, Diksha, Kevin O'Fallon, Priscilla M. Clarkson, C. Patrick Dunne, Karen R. Conca, and Bozena Michniak-Kohn. "Comparison of Quercetin Pharmacokinetics Following Oral Supplementation in Humans." *Journal of Food Science* 77, no. 11 (2012): H231–38.

Kodack, Marc. *Fully Burdened Cost of Managing Waste in Contingency Operations.* Arlington, VA: Army Environmental Policy Institute, 2011.

Lavigne, Peter, Zach Patterson, Shubman Chandra, Derek Affonce, Karen Benedek, and Phil Carbone. *Controlling Ethylene for Extended Preservation of Fresh Fruit and Vegetables.* Fort Belvoir, VA: Defense Technical Information Center, 2009.

Lee, Thomas Ming-Hung. "Over-the-Counter Biosensors: Past, Present, and Future." *Sensors* 8, no. 9 (2008): 5535–59.

"Maersk Container Industry Is Partnering with Primaira LLC to Develop an Air Cleaning System in Star Cool Integrated Refrigerated Containers." *Food Logistics,* January 31, 2014. Accessed June 26, 2014. http://www.foodlogistics.com/news/11302738/maersk-container-industry-is-partnering-with-primaira-llc-to-develop-an-air-cleaning-system-in-star-cool-integrated-refrigerated-containers.

Massachusetts Institute of Technology. Proctor Papers, MC 0268. Institute Archives and Special Collections, MIT Libraries, Cambridge, MA.

Moody, Stephen. Interview by the author, July 9, 2014.

Operational Rations of the Department of Defense. 9th ed. Natick, MA: U.S. Army Natick Soldier Research, Development and Engineering Center, 2012.

Peake, Libby. "Puzzling Over Incineration." *Resource Magazine,* December 16, 2013. Accessed February 2014. http://www.resource.uk.com/article/Techniques _Innovation/Puzzling_over_incineration.

Petrovick, Martha S., James D. Harper, Frances E. Nargi, Eric D. Schwoebel, Mark C. Hennessy, Todd H. Rider, and Mark A. Hollis. "Rapid Sensors for Biological-Agent Identification." *Lincoln Laboratory Journal* 17, no. 1 (2007): 63–84.

PWTB 200-1-83: Feasibility of JP-8 Recycling at Fort Bragg, NC. Washington, DC: U.S. Army Corps of Engineers, 2010.

Ruppert, W. H. *Force Provider Solid Waste Characterization Study.* Fort Belvoir, VA: Defense Technical Information Center, 2004.

Sudarsky, Jerry. "Jerry Sudarsky: Wasco Scientist and International Humanitarian." Interview by Gilbert Gia, Bakersfield, CA, 2008. Accessed December 11, 2014. http://www.gilbertgia.com/hist_articles/people/Sudarsky_invent_peo2.pdf.

Valdes, James J., Darrel E. Menking, and Mia Paterno, eds. *Third Annual Conference on Receptor-Based Biosensors.* Aberdeen Proving Ground, MD: U.S. Army Armaments Munitions Chemical Command, 1988.

Wiesner, Jerome B. *Vannevar Bush, 1890–1974: A Biographical Memoir.* Washington, DC: National Academy of Sciences, 1979.

Wilson, Charles L. *Intelligent and Active Packaging for Fruits and Vegetables.* Boca Raton, FL: CRC Press, 2007.

CHAPTER 14. DO WE REALLY WANT OUR CHILDREN EATING LIKE SPECIAL OPS?

"Administrative Law—Regulatory Design—Food Safety Modernization Act Implements Private Regulatory Scheme—FDA Food Safety Modernization Act." *Harvard Law Review* 125, no. 3 (2012): 859–66.

Bedard, Kelly. "The Long-Term Impact of Military Service on Health: Evidence from World War II and Korean War Veterans." *American Economic Review* 96, no. 1 (2006): 176–94.

Degnan, Frederick H. "Emerging Technologies and Their Implications: Where Policy, Science, and Law Intersect." *Food and Drug Law Journal* 53, no. 4 (1998): 593–96.

Eisenbrand, Gerhard. "Safety Assessment of High Pressure Treated Foods." Presentation at German Research Foundation, Senate Commission for Food Safety, November 21, 2005. Downloaded April 5, 2014. http://www.dfg.de/download/pdf/ dfg_im_profil/reden_stellungnahmen/2005/sklm_high_pressure_2005_en.pdf.

Elder, G. H., E. C. Clipp, J. S. Brown, L. R. Martin, and H. S. Friedman. "The Lifelong Mortality Risks of World War II Experiences." *Research on Aging* 31, no. 4 (2009): 391–412.

Freeman, Marilyn M. "Providing Technology Enabled Capabilities." Paper presented at the 12th Annual Science & Engineering Technology Conference/DOD Tech Exposition, Department of Defense, Washington, DC, June 22, 2011.

Hahn, Martin J. "FDA Has the Legal Authority to Adopt a Threshold of Toxicological Concern (TTC) for Substances in Food at Trace Levels." *Food and Drug Law Journal* 65, no. 2 (2010): 217–30.

Kokini, Jozef. Interview by the author, February 26, 2011.

Lykken, Sara. "We Really Need to Talk: Adapting FDA Processes to Rapid Change." *Food and Drug Law Journal* 68, no. 4 (2013): 357–400.

McNally, David. "Future Soldiers Will Have Flexible Electronics Everywhere." States News Service, February 19, 2013.

Maxwell, David S. "Thoughts on the Future of Special Operations." *Small Wars Journal* 9, no. 10, October 31, 2013.

Rodricks, Joseph V. "Assessing and Managing Health Risks from Chemical Constituents and Contaminants of Food." Paper presented at the Workshop on a Framework for Assessing the Health, Environmental and Social Effects of the Food System, the Institute of Medicine, Washington, DC, September 16, 2013.

Soldier 2025: New Technologies Anticipated for the Future Warfighter. Natick, MA: U.S. Army Natick Soldier Research, Development and Engineering Center, 2000.

Sustainable Forward Operating Bases. Falls Church, VA: Strategic Environmental Research and Development Program, 2010.

Vine, David. "The Pentagon's New Generation of Secret Military Bases." *Mother Jones,* July 16, 2012.

Index